MONSTER

MONSTER

JENEVA BURROUGHS STONE

for Robert

and for the readers of
Busily Seeking ... Continual Change

ACKNOWLEDGEMENTS

Eternal gratitude to Eleanor Wilner for the use of her home to write, her encouragement, and her careful reading of this manuscript over time. Thanks to Sarah Manguso, Elizabeth Aquino, Blase Reardon, and April Ossmann for reading this manuscript in its various forms. Special thanks to my husband Roger, to Heather McHugh for taking care of the caregivers, and to C. Jimmy Lin and Rare Genomics Institute.

The seed for this manuscript was "The Chaos," which both Daisy Fried and Karen Brennan read and critiqued at the Warren Wilson MFA Program—much gratitude to both of them. Thanks also to both the *30/30 Project* at *Tupelo Press* and to Daisy Fried's *24PearlStreet* workshop, during which six of these poems were generated.

Finally, I am grateful for the support of the MacDowell and Millay Colonies, which gave me time and space to write, as well as meaningful connections to other artists.

—

Gracious acknowledgement to the following journals for their support by publishing these works:

"Winter Kept Us Warm" in *Colorado Review*; "The Brain as Variation" in *Poetry International* (UCSD) as "The Brain as Variation (or a Theme)"; "In which I am envious of the Eternal" in *Pleiades* as "In which I am envious of the Eternal (Ezekiel?) and say so"; "Oscillation" in *Orphan Diseases in the Age of Health 2.0* as "Rte. 125"; "After Life" in *Poet Lore*; "The Chaos" in *qarrtsiluni* as "Female Parent"; "Meiosis" in *Waxwing*; "Notes on Creativity & Originality" in *jmww*; "Disability & Space-Time Considerations" in *New England Review Digital*.

Pieces of "Commonplaces" first appeared in *EDNA* as "Our Bodies Are Our Temples" and in *The Collagist* as "That I May See Thee."

Pieces of "Altimeter" first appeared in *LARB* as "Still to Behold, Still to Be Told," and in *Tupelo Quarterly* as "Radio Silence."

Contents

monster, *n., adv., and adj.*

Etymology: < Anglo-Norman and Middle French *monstre, moustre,* French *monstre* (mid 12th cent. in Old French as *mostre* in sense "prodigy, marvel", first half of the 13th cent. in senses "disfigured person" and "misshapen being", c1223 in extended sense applied to a pagan, first half of the 18th cent. by antiphrasis denoting an extraordinarily attractive thing) < classical Latin *mōnstrum* portent, prodigy, monstrous creature, wicked person, monstrous act, atrocity < the base of *monēre* to warn.

A2. *n.*
Something extraordinary or unnatural; an amazing event or occurrence; a prodigy, a marvel. *Obs.*

C2. *adj.*
colloq. Outstanding, extraordinarily good; remarkably successful.

—Oxford English Dictionary, 3rd ed.

Holocene

One day my child stared, watching his brain chemicals dance. He then tried to crawl; I have never seen motion broken down into so many pieces, never seen a world shatter like ice.

> *(The Buddhist nun who blessed him wrote*
> *once how she held the begging bowl, realizing*
> *her lesson: possibilities open when I let go of what*
> *I think I want—the energy of grasping, a barrier.)*

Pouring water into a broken bowl might resemble the act of loving: with each attempt to cover cracks, some slips away. The same might be said of mercy—that humankind can never hold enough, even in a million outstretched hands.

> *(We watched him drawn through the cold,*
> *white O of the CT scan—that morning he'd*
> *looked at arms and hands in turn before he*
> *changed, expressions shaken silk across his face.)*

The world can suddenly buckle and tear because nature tends toward destruction (earthquakes, floods, winds and snow). But I fear love will be the force that breaks me.

> *(As a child, I saw the aurora borealis,*
> *pale green silk wavering in the dark, but*
> *once it was the right kind of cold, the aurora*
> *vibrant with fingers of pink, blue and white.)*

I lived north then, where the first snow filled us with delight. Things happen for a reason, they say—the change of seasons, health and disease, our shifting climate, love and hope and the course of life.

Yet sometimes what happens breaks covenant with every explanation in its path, the heart ground slowly into rubble under advancing ice, while the aurora shimmers forth its false embrace.

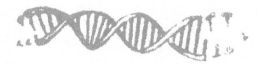

Winter Kept Us Warm

The day I was married, it snowed.

When I woke, I could see only blurred sky. But I knew. When it snows or is about to snow, the air has a quality to it like the inside of a steel canister. The world closes in and the atmosphere becomes metallic.

Snow in November was not, in and of itself, unusual—especially in Vermont, where the wedding took place. I wore Maine hunting boots under my wedding dress to the old meetinghouse where we said our vows, the snow adding to the general excitement. An event, the way the brightness of snow covers what, in contrast, appears dark—the ordinary become the unexpected.

My graduate school roommate told me that, in some Asian cultures, snow is considered a sign of luck.

And luck is out of our control.

—

A friend once mentioned that skiers often say, "Turn in the white, miss the black." He heard it while skiing the backcountry out West, an old burn area, all black charred trunks rising up against a downhill slope of clean snow. Moving through this, the black and white flicker became disorienting, and he said he had to look for white—focus on the spaces, not the obstacles—to maintain control.

For a while, this became my mantra, *turn in the white, miss the black,* look for the white spaces, ignore the obstacles. The flicker of escape in rapid interstitial intersection with dark reality.

—

When I first learned I was pregnant, I was alone. Staring at the lines on the white test strip, a sense of awe settled over me—an awe like the flash before fear rushes dark into that bright opening. I sat down at our dining table pondering the weight of this responsibility. I kept my misgivings to myself.

I gave birth to a child who seemed typical at first, but who, thirteen months into his life, crashed through a weakened floor in the house of his being in a catastrophic medical event. He was left profoundly disabled. We didn't know what triggered his collapse and he remained undiagnosed for fourteen years.

—

I can remember, as a child in Vermont, snow banks higher than myself lining the walkway that led from our front porch to the sidewalk, and the snow on my grandparents' farm obliterating every mark of normalcy, changing our landmarks. All this disorientation a form of play: the known world inverted, the ordinary become the unexpected.

Winter in the DC area, where I now live, isn't much, most of the time: the occasional huge snowfall, smatterings of ice and slush, and so on. An inconvenience, really. My daughter (my second child) loves these brief glimpses of winter. A look through a glass darkly into another world, I suppose.

But my son, Robert, now wheelchair-bound, can't navigate the outdoors in a foot or two of snow. So when the big storms come, we're confined to the house. Trapped might be another word for it.

I have come to prefer spring.

—

An old memory, a non sequitur, declares itself repeatedly: I'm driving my cousin Amelia into Burlington in my parents' car, and we're headed around a moderate curve. Amelia is very young, perhaps six or seven—a serious child with close-cropped dark hair—she is strapped into the passenger seat. I may be in high school or even college, and I've had a driver's license from the time I was 14 years old.

It is snowing, or it has been snowing, and there is a light accumulation on the road and the shoulders. Maybe I hit the brake lightly, or maybe it's a consequence of the dynamics of steering, but the car goes into a gentle skid. Amelia has been quiet, as she usually is, but her voice pitches high and startled, "We're slidin'!"

And we *are* sliding several feet to the side of the road. I learned to drive before anti-lock brakes were standard, so I have undoubtedly released my foot from the brake and am steering into the skid with the wheels locked and that ineffective feeling of the steering wheel rotating far too lightly in my hands.

———

I know an avalanche researcher: winter his favorite season in all its beauty and danger. He reminds me that the qualities of snow are not uniform: crystals vary in size and structure, from the large fluffy snowflakes of children's picture books to the smaller ones that cluster in a blizzard, to the hard nubbins of sleet. The different waxes for cross country skis reflect this: icy, granular, soft powder, heavy and wet snow. Thus, snow has personality—as Wilson "Snowflake" Bentley argued, no two snowflakes are alike. And no two snowfalls, perhaps, either.

Weather conditions—humidity and sun and wind—affect mountain slopes where snow gathers pristine white against a sharp blue sky. With each storm, snow accumulates in different layers. Sometimes one of the layers is thin and weak, or unstable, like cake crumbs shifting in a box between the hard pack of the storms before and after it. An avalanche is triggered when the weight of the upper layers puts stress on the weak layer, and, thus, these snow stacks, invisible to the casual observer, collapse and slide, often with catastrophic results.

When a person is trapped in an avalanche, death comes most often by suffocation. The weight and torque of the rapidly shearing snow envelop the skier, filling the nose and mouth, pinning or splaying the limbs, and settling in a snowpack that sets like cement, the skier's arms and legs isolated and useless.

———

Nothing happens. Amelia is probably frightened, but shrugs it off when I tell her we're OK. After all, she's old enough now to grasp that floating feeling cars have on snow sometimes, as the wheels slide just within the driver's control, shimmying on the snow the way you might feel on skis before kicking off and gliding.

The steering wheel now gone heavy with traction, I pull the car back onto the main roadbed and we continue on our way.

—

Sick children are often said to "declare" themselves when their bodies announce an intention to carry on with this life.

I don't remember exactly when or how Robert declared himself during the low point of his initial illness. I can remember his body curling inward as it looked like he would round the curve toward coma. But I was determined that he stay and I felt my mind trying to attach itself to his to prevent his leaving. He never slid away completely, and his spirit gained traction bit by bit as he pulled—or I pulled him—back to a facsimile of consciousness. His body, though, slid away into disability, frantic, tumbling, over the course of a few days.

—

The winter of 2010, after two storms hit within one week, leaving more than thirty inches of snow, the DC metro area was declared a disaster area. People here throw up their hands at snow and retreat into their homes as though the day of judgment were near. School is canceled, the federal government goes on its liberal leave policy, the plows don't hit your neighborhood for days. Local and state governments repeatedly tell us that all hope is lost, we will be alone, the power company cannot be expected to be held responsible for keeping the lights on, the area will be shut down indefinitely, call us in the spring.

—

When I was young, my parents believed in mastering snow. Snow tires, chains, learning the gradual rocking acceleration, forward and reverse, required to dislodge a stuck tire. All of this perfectly ordinary. Ordinary that my father would drive forty miles to pick me up from college for the weekend during the middle of a storm that dropped at least eighteen inches. That we would take the back roads home because Route 7 was too slippery with traffic and compressed ice. That all would be well until we faced the road on the big hill south of Monkton, its blacktop gone, its edges only faint indentations. That he would turn to me and say, "Well, at least we've got the downhill to accelerate—rear wheel drive will push us up!" And it did, the late-model Cadillac shimmying a bit on the front end.

Accelerate slow and steady. Keep your speed even. Use low gear.

———

In the evening after the first big storm that frosted the DC area like a white cake, I went outside and crossed the street to deliver a meal to a neighbor who needed it. Returning through the middle of our road, I paused in the knee-deep tire ruts left by the handful of four-wheel-drive urban warriors who'd passed through. Looked up the street, looked down. Absorbed the pleasure of standing in the middle—though ours is not a busy street—without a worry or a thought about a car's approach. Streetlights made the snow glow in a blue-white haze that settled over all.

There is a peace that follows disaster of some sort—perhaps the quieting of all inner voices, all the chatter layered onto the days, whether people or cars or planes or the frenetic over-scheduling and task overload. All of that tamped down under two feet of snow.

And yet. The snow that winter was a relief, an odd blessing. A transformation from one state to another, or a reminder that transformation was possible. The unexpected become the ordinary.

Locked up in our home, together, there seemed little to fear. Our power was on. We had food. All of Robert's medical supplies were in good order. No reason to leave the house until the plow came—and even then, no reason to leave until the high-pitched hunting and gathering post-storm fray had subsided.

Calm. Until that winter, snowstorms had provoked anxiety and fear in me. I thought of myself as "trapped" in the house, my disabled child sick, his health always uncertain.

———

My son's collapse was so sudden, so unexpected; it came without a single warning. Throughout the fourteen years before diagnosis, one neurologist never ruled out the possibility of an underlying

9

metabolic disorder. A metabolic disorder is triggered when a child's increasing weight, his body mass, outstrips the compromised ability of the body's biochemical processes. A faltering metabolic process, one misstep in a chain of manufacture and reaction, results in a cascade of motor and cognitive malfunctions that build like a pile of talus at the base of a slope.

One of Robert's symptoms was global ataxia, or the body's inability to control and coordinate the movements of muscles, and, therefore, limbs—as though his body were divided into four separate containers or cells, one for each limb. My earliest observations were that each of his arms and each of his legs moved separately. One hand might approach the imaginary plane that bisected his face and chest, but stop just short, as though the hand had encountered an invisible barrier. The other would be unable to meet it. Each isolated and useless.

I could bring my hands together, and late at night, I closed myself in the bathroom, alone, knelt at the white edge of the tub and prayed. This, too, I kept to myself.

———

Christmas Eve is the night the world often seems to stand still—a long night of waiting and arrival after a day of frenetic activity. Streets empty and lights dimmed. The night the world declares itself. And the night my new year always begins.

My adolescent memories of Christmas Eve involve driving to midnight services, the halting fall of snow flurries whiter and brighter against the black around us, flickering like a photonegative—white then black, superimposed, disorienting. Yet the car always carries us safely around the curve on which Amelia and I skidded. Sometimes the roads are clear, the smooth whoosh of blacktop beneath us; sometimes the tires are muffled, the treads lifting and tossing the snow, the barest tension of traction. The minister reading from the scripture Mary's reaction to the shepherds, *But Mary kept all these things, pondering them in her heart.* Her response to this the same as to her pregnancy: sober and awed at what has been revealed to her. What she cannot change, nor speak of.

—

In the months that followed the onset of Robert's illness, I found myself pregnant again, accidentally. The emotional intensity of those days is blinding, returning to them like coming out of a dark tunnel into the supernova of noon sunlight on a snow-covered landscape.

On three successive nights during that pregnancy, I had three dreams. I've never had dreams like these before or since; in fact, I rarely dream at all anymore. Describing them to anyone always feels crazy because they were all of the same texture, all three, and it was a single dream in three parts, a triptych. In the first, a blond child who appeared to be Robert started walking again. In the second, the same child started talking. In the third, I miscarried.

I woke each morning to a sense of disorientation: the dream world had been capaciously real, as though I had walked into another room of my life, a room in which everything was just as it should be, not as it was. And yet I woke into the known world each day, confused by the flicker between the two, between what could be and what is.

The only way to reconcile this was to look for the interstices— to believe the future was being imparted to me, and it would not be unhappy.

I held those dreams close to my heart for years without telling anyone except my husband. They were an arrival, an annunciation, a declaration, the present and the future sliding together the way the brain perceives objects in the midst of a skid: at times, you are sliding toward the tree, at other times, the tree is rushing toward you.

I did miscarry a few days after the third dream. And, eventually, as I continued to believe these were a truth shared with me, I understood that the child in the dreams was not Robert with his brown hair, but my daughter, Edith, who was born a year and a half later with a full head of bright white-blond hair.

—

As the snow was plowed that winter, pushed back into monstrous twelve-foot piles in parking lots, in front of sidewalks, at the corners of intersections, Edith took to calling them the Alps. Climbing the Alps became one of her favorite activities.

We have pictures of her and her brother posed in front of these craggy mounds of snow—the two of them small and delighted, oblivious to the mock threat of the shoved and tumbled snow behind them, blackened at its edges with soot. Robert's wheelchair arrayed like green blades bright against the near-white snow.

The truth is, that winter was the first time we thought of Robert's disabilities as permanent. For years, his abilities—to eat, to speak, to walk, to use his hands and fingers—flickered in ways that now seem indescribable as dreams. A hazy syllable there, increased stepping reflex here. An ability to grasp, for a few days, an object between thumb and finger. An intermittent opportunity to cleanly select items on a communication device, a constellation of motions that would surface, disappear, then re-surface for years. Each of these returning periodically like random green shoots through an early spring snow.

In another set of photos, Robert, my husband and my daughter pose, wedged narrowly between snow banks higher than the kids, on the dark surface of the freshly shoveled walkway in front of our house. Robert is not afraid, even though every mark of normalcy, most landmarks, are gone, the rims of his wheelchair scraping the snow stacks.

When I look at these pictures, I think about our known world inverted. How ordinary this all seems: my daughter mugging for the camera, my son smiling in his wheelchair, the handicapped ramp and its pale yellow railing a fixture I notice only because the static flicker of its many posts and balusters is trellised with snow.

———

To a friend who had suffered a great loss, I wrote what I then believed to be true: that control of our lives is an illusion. I was not surprised when she agreed.

It would be easy to say, *an illusion as temporal as snow.* I don't know if I believe it to be true. In the heart of winter, we may become uncertain spring will resurface, pulling with cruel force an unreal city of crocus and daffodil from the brown-fogged earth. But the fact of snow remains, dazzling as crystals scattered in our hair, accumulating in the interstices of a world we thought we knew.

—

At Christmas this year, my daughter, my father and I went walking in the snow around the perimeter of what I'll probably always call my grandparents" farm, even though the two of them are gone. Four to five inches of completely white, mostly untracked snow covered the meadows and rock outcroppings and decaying farm tools, but it was not enough to bury last summer's three-foot dry stalks of Queen Anne's lace and goldenrod extending upward from the brightening field.

Sometimes the snow declares itself with wind, or mixed with sleet, taps its fingernails lightly on the windowpane. But in the Vermont of my childhood, the snow mostly arrived unannounced, as if by chance—it is, really, the snow that comes in on little cat feet, not the fog. Awakening on those mornings to that sense of white bright disorientation, I opened my eyes to a world transformed.

My cousin Amelia and I are, once again, passengers in the same car— her daughter, born prematurely, is at a children's hospital in Boston. Natalie is slowly pulling herself through the complications of an early birth, some of which will be lasting, while a rare chromosomal disorder makes itself manifest.

And the future and the past are sliding toward us or we toward them, each of us with our hands on the wheel, pretending to steer toward the white spaces and, some days, feeling the heaviness of traction.

Commonplaces

I once attended a lecture by a famous poet. She delivered an intelligent and carefully composed speech in which she analogized something about poetry with the development of speech in children. I don't remember the connection she drew to poetry because I could focus only on her assertion that the ability to speak, to process the world into language, is the primary turning point for a child, what makes a child fully human at last. I left, puzzled.

Maybe she meant "originality" in poetic diction makes poetry real? Language gives rise to an innate, original being? Or that, without language, a person could be no more than a product of gestation and the accidents of genetic recombination? My son was in elementary school. It was common for teachers and other parents to believe his physically compromised body (he doesn't speak) meant he had a limited intelligence or none at all.

In *Explorata: Or Discoveries*, his commonplace book on language and rhetoric, Ben Jonson writes, "Language most shows a man: speak that I may see thee. It springs out of the most retired, and inmost parts of us, and is the image of the parent of it, the mind."

These are not Jonson's original thoughts. A commonplace book—a Renaissance cultural practice—was used to jot down bits of prose or poetry by others, or observations on those. Jonson often elaborated on the work of other writers as he saw fit. Here, he translates Erasmus, *oratio imago animi*, "speech is the image of the soul," or "speak that I may see thee," and remixes those thoughts with his own, and those of Quintilian and Cicero.

Each time I re-read, I'm struck by Jonson's observation that language has a parent—the mind. Words are child-like transcriptions.

—

At the age of two, my son stopped taking food and liquid by mouth—he ate and drank, very feebly, for a year after an undiagnosed breakdown. We spent two hours or more on each meal. One little bit of feta cheese to the lips, push it in, see if he could swallow it.

Robert did not gain any weight for a year, and he barely grew in height and head circumference. One day, at the end of a long week spending most days trying to get food in him at all, he stopped eating altogether.

Moving to artificial food intake, nasogastric then gastric tube-feeding, was psychologically difficult for us, although it saved Robert's life. The bright reds of tomatoes, the texture of rice, the colors and shapes of other foods were still there for us, and visible to him, but the substance was gone, replaced with an oily, thick formula the unpleasant smell of which was covered up with artificial flavoring, that odor that tries too hard to be something it's not.

What food meant changed. For Robert it became the language of his birth, now foreign to him. For my husband and myself, cooking became a late-evening ritual we performed with care once Robert was settled, as parents spell words so their children will not understand.

—

Pregnant with Robert, I taught Jonson's poem, "On My First Son," which eulogizes his namesake:

> Rest in soft peace, and, asked, say here doth lie
> Ben Jonson his best piece of poetry.
> For whose sake, henceforth, all his vows be such,
> As what he loves may never like too much.

Note the seamless merging of filial and parental identity, split in agony by the last line—that such a distinction between like and love might exist. The line, though, isn't Jonson's. Martial is its parent: *quidquid ames; cupids non placuisse nimis*, "whatever you love, pray that you do not find it too pleasing."

I did not take the last line as a warning.

Our bodies are our temples, runs a commonplace of modern thought, and if we don't nourish ourselves properly during pregnancy, or our infants optimally after birth, we might damage their brain development. We must eat even those foods we dislike while expecting, for the nutritional value. So much for "you are what you eat": most women hope for a child they will like, who will be like them. "A healthy baby."

My maternal body had ingested gametes and delivered with complexity of thought, a child. People speak of the process of thinking as "digesting information" or gestating ideas, and so the brain's byproducts, thought and speech, can be expressed in abstractions that link eating and thinking and, also, child-bearing: ingestion, consumption, composition, gestation, digestion, elimination.

—

In a brightly lit hospital room, we're happy, because the nasogastric tube has animated Robert's frame. He's getting enough calories and fluid and he's lively and interested in the world around him again. A bright yellow tube is taped to his cheek and snakes into his nose and from there to his esophagus and stomach.

He's talking—saying a few words, or fragments of words. We have a plush wind-up frog with which we are amusing him, and he's saying "-ggie," "-ggie." He also says a garbled phrase, which he repeats enough that we can untangle the sounds and realize he's saying, "I love you."

The small cache of English and invented words he'd drawn together by the age of one were missing, but not gone, the net loosed and the words floating like deep-water fish in the depths of his consciousness.

So we are ecstatic. Within a few weeks, though, this ability recedes. We never know why.

—

Talking and eating appear to be distinct activities: the first an indicator of intelligence, controlled by the higher functions of the brain, and the second an animal function so basic that even brainless organisms like sponges, coral and bacteria have openings to gulp and ingest food. Robert could do neither, yet he had things to tell us. While liquid pumped into his stomach, gestures broke the surface of his mind's pool: eye gaze, smile, the varied pitch of cries, the contortions of his face.

For most people, speaking and eating are two sides of the same coin, an output and an input, respectively, of the mouth and throat muscles. Speech therapists categorize basic language as ins and outs: receptive and expressive, what a child understands and what a child can communicate. Receptive skills are hard to gauge, murky, like our early attempts to measure how much food Robert ingested and how much he spat out. Expressive language, however, can show off the talents of the tiniest gourmets, whether their alimentary aptitude rises to the diction of shrimp scampi, or stops at peanut butter and jelly.

The mind, behind the scenes, gestates language, "makes the man," so to speak. Jonson continues thus, "No glass renders a man's form, or likeness, so true as his speech. Nay, it is likened to a man: and as we consider feature, and composition in a man; so words in language: in the greatness, aptness, sound, structure, and harmony of it."

Renaissance poets liked that analogy, *you are what you say*.

—

I am certain Robert understands what's said to him. In fact, listening is his most critical sensory in-route. When his eyes can't follow, when his body stays in place, his hearing, a purse-seine, gathers up the room, catching brightly flickering words like fish, and reeling them in.

Think about pushing a button in order to communicate, or choosing among two or four buttons. Every day, many of us make this motion over and over again: elevator buttons, doorbells, computer keys, blender buttons. Some of these targets are small, some are large. Few of us think about it, but the ability to press buttons or choose among keys rests on an ability to make all of the micro-motions described above. Fluidly and without thought.

Robert finds all of these difficult or impossible on any given day. Even with the help of devices for the disabled, like large red switches, six inches in diameter, that depress with the slightest touch, or in-line communicators angled upward at 30 degrees with colored square keys that require just the corner pushed down, he can barely sustain the effort.

Touch-screen computer-driven devices are out because he drags his hand as he moves it, if he can move it. Even now, I am still briefly flustered if I press the wrong key on my computer and the whole screen changes. Drag the hand across a touch screen and unintended words come to the fore.

Still, he likes the in-line communicator with its four buttons I can record for him. Each button says something to which another person can respond: I love you, I need some love, I am Superman, Look at me, *Hola* everyone, and so on. He likes this ability to say something, even if it may not be what is actually on his mind, even if he continues to be the kid behind the curtain of my voice.

In his own time, Jonson was most famous for his plays, distinctive voices in dialogue.

—

I have only ever been dis-abled during labor. A permanent concave curl in my lower back, a souvenir of carrying in front, is all that's left to remind me. When contractions started in earnest, I realized the inanity of pregnancy books claiming breathing exercises and talismans like music and a favorite nightie would put me in charge. This process would own me.

Before an epidural could be administered, my field of vision narrowed to tiny circles while a white-brightness burst in sparks from the center outward. My body became concentric, contractions radiating from back to front and front to back, in an unstoppable process of elimination. Robert didn't descend properly, and, by the end, my vaginal canal served as stage for an amphitheater of nurses, residents and my obstetrician. An episiotomy ensued, followed by an intervention with a suction device, a warning about an emergency C-section, and then Robert came through at the last possible moment with the help of forceps. My blood loss was significant enough that my husband said I turned pale green.

My most vivid memory remains staring, late at night, at a cup of juice and three saltines set a few inches from me on a table, my audience dispersed, even my husband sleeping soundly. I hadn't eaten in over 24 hours. My blood couldn't carry enough oxygen so I could raise my arm to reach the food or my voice to summon anyone.

Robert, however, was fine—red and bawling, his Apgar scores nines.

—

Late-night TV ads voice alarm over "birth accidents" the same way these claims attorneys speak of automobile collisions: sudden, unknown, unavoidable. Disaster can strike in the form of oxygen deprivation at birth, but brain, nerve and muscle cells may be compromised at any moment from the earliest stages of fetal development to the end of life because they respire via biochemical and electron chains, the lungs only a pump, the body's cells working from the instruction template they've been given by DNA. But we sue to compensate for our losses, our differences only when we could not have been responsible.

People assume responsible pregnancies are intentional, the act of making a child thought out thoroughly. My obstetrician compares the reproductive instinct to salmon swimming upstream, lemmings rushing over a cliff—a primal feeling overriding the rational mind. So much for the mind's attempts at parenting. During sex most people lose facility with language.

In the end, one can become a reflection of what one eats, treat the body as a temple, spin like a politician the humble wish for "just a healthy baby," but the body will own us, each and every one. That is, one can form a responsible intention to have a child, but no one biologically gestates an idea.

—

I write poems and essays about my son. Childishly, I believe I can convey my son's essence to someone else by using words common to us all. I can dress him and decorate him as any parent would, but his mind will be his own. I can make a character of him as in a play, channeling his personality through my words, but his original script remains backstage.

Jonson says, "Language most shows a man: speak that I may see thee," but what does he mean by language? Words? Maybe—but he writes to explain what the Ancients meant by rhetorical style: high, middle, plain, low. The method, the ornamentation, not the substance—the means of communication and not the exact diction.

For example, I could say that Jonson translates or copies or channels Erasmus, but all I mean to say is that whatever the words flickering between the two men, as each speaks for the other, something of each becomes visible.

Speak that I may *see* thee.

Robert's most reliable and available communication strategy: to raise his right arm for yes, his left for no. At times, we must look for even the slightest shift in either limb. Every once in a while my mimetic curtain parts and he is there, himself.

Brain as Variation

The world is briefly frozen in place. Otherwise, it would fly apart. I cut a fennel bulb in half this evening, in between the stalks and through the center. From a triangular core, the strata of the plant piles in convex layers outward and then upward in shoots and fronds. I thought about whether it looked like a brain, and the nub of the core like a brainstem. And when the core was removed, the layers fell apart and scattered like beach shells.

The last week has scattered a bit like that. The weekend shapes up and it looks as though the parts of the week will cohere, perhaps not in a linear, day by day fashion, but at least as a series of overlapping events and connections. Then there are snow days and the core falls out, and the children and the laundry and the email and the work projects end up disconnected and scattered.

When I must make excuses for things left undone, I tell people I have a disabled child. A label of convenience, this acts as an adhesive strip to briefly secure his discordant pieces: no speech, tube-fed, wheelchair-bound, lively eyes. I don't say, Robert developed typically until he was one, or has been undiagnosed for many years. People like labels; they don't know how to tie off loose threads.

I learned recently that the basal ganglia is the brain's clearinghouse: the world gives it information piecemeal, which it sorts and routes to other parts of the brain for analysis, and the analysis is delivered back to it for speech and action. When the basal ganglia doesn't function properly, information, memories, and impressions scatter. Robert's basal ganglia is damaged.

———

I read the first poem in Ron Silliman's *The Alphabet* last week, and am still mulling my response to it. Its title is "Albany," a place close to where I grew up, a place I've never visited, only driven through or around via the box of highways that joins I-87, the Northway, and I-90 west to Buffalo or east to Boston.

It's a prose poem, and its method is disjuncture. So, like anything postmodern I've loved, David Antin or Anne Carson or Lyn Hejinian, you move both forward in the time-space that is reading, and also to the center and back out again. This latter motion is like a transportation hub, in that thoughts like vehicles move inward and outward along key phrases, but it's also threading a needle and sewing. Thoughts are thread that loops through an opening, and a good stitch moves forward, but then hooks back through the trail of its own passing.

Perpetually back-stepping, I don't feel led to a conclusion, and I don't feel as though everything must be in order. My mind is freed to wander among the sentences, the ideas, the images, and enter the work from the front door or the back, or the window, if I find that opening most accessible.

—

David Antin says, "i choose it [the label "poet," as opposed to another type of artist] in spite of the fact that i tend to feel a little uncomfortable with it because if im going to be a poet i want to be a poet who explores mind as the medium of his poetry   not mind as a static thing   but the act of thinking and the closest i can come to the act of thinking is the act of talking and thinking at the same time."

The idea of "mind" as the medium of poetry suggests thought as movement, which sets up an inevitable question, I suppose: whether the mind can be static, or what aspect of "mind" Antin sees as static, as, say, a neurologist might see it. I worry that neurologists do see the mind as static, or perhaps they don't differentiate between "mind" and "brain"—they see the world in terms of brains that are damaged or undamaged, processes that are normal or abnormal. I don't know that they see fluidity among states. But of course, to me, as to Antin, the mind is fluid, developing, shifting—never truly stopped or still. Moving language, "talk," as the opposite of "page" stasis, is what Antin means, I think. Capturing those patterns of energy, of kinesis.

—

We feel constantly defeated in so many ways by Robert's disabilities because of this mythic disabled child we hear so much about from those who monitor such things: doctors, therapists, educators. This child who rises from a fixed point of disability and grows from that place. The child whose disabilities are "stabilized." Does that kid exist?

From the outside looking in, many people see disability as a fixed point on a spectrum of abilities: as whatever it is that your child cannot do, or where your child appears to be located on the sliding scale of relative achievement and ability that other parents use to measure their own children. But, of course, (childhood) disability is not a fixed point—even Christopher Reeve gave the lie to the idea that paralysis is a juncture at which a human being is forever stuck, like a butterfly on a pin in a display case.

As when the neurologist draws a line graph and explains Robert's "aspect" to us: *Some kids who come to us,* he says, *have been developing like this* (he draws a diagonal line upward from the zero/zero coordinates), *but then this happens* (he draws a sharp downward angle). *Sometimes, they recover* (up goes the line again). *Others develop for a little while* (on the upward diagonal) *and then just level out* (he draws a straight line to the edge of the graph). *Kids in Robert's medical spectrum look like this*—and he draws a squiggly line moving up and away from zero/zero, but dipping and rising and not on a steady diagonal. The back and forth represents losses and gains and regains and losses again, but all at different coordinates; nothing that is gained or lost has any equivalency.

This is how I know I can trust this neurologist. Even in the years before I knew Robert's basal ganglia was faulty, I used this metaphor: his mind and brain, his mental and physical abilities, are like a multi-faceted crystal globe rotated against a light source. Some weeks, certain facets refract the light spectrum and glitter their colors. Then the globe rotates in another direction and those abilities recede and other facets are brightly lit.

No one understood my metaphor. But this neurologist does. Our metaphors are the same, mathematic, geometrical, but taking variant shapes.

—

On my desk at work there are several pictures of each of my children—school pictures from the last few years. My attention is drawn repeatedly to the difference between Robert's 4th grade and his 5th grade pictures.

In his 4th grade picture, Robert's face is still full: his cheeks are round and childish. In his 5th grade picture, his jaw line is longer, his face has thinned out a bit. He still looks the child, but is taking on the contours of adolescence. I confess he looks very handsome. I also confess that I don't know how to move forward from here.

For most of Robert's life, my role has been restricted to helping him endure some sort of medical protocol that I would rather he not have. But I put on my cheery or my empathetic or my comforting face, knowing all the while that I am being asked to lie. Because it is going to hurt or it's not going to be pleasant or I have to believe someone else myself that this procedure really is going to make a difference. So I am often the Angel of False Comfort, shrinking mentally behind what a "parent" is apparently supposed to do: comfort her child under any and all circumstances and say it will be alright.

This creates a sort of distance: here I am in my body, just fine; but there he is in his body, not so fine, the body that I made myself for him. He is me and not me.

—

Language, lies, language—a series of signs, a forest of representation, the endless attempt to close the gap between *res* and *verba*. There are people who believe only in things and feel language to be a lie.

24

There are people who believe that only language exists and exists to articulate a world that is an illusion. Then there are people like me, sitting in a small boat in the middle of a lake, wanting to row toward two shores simultaneously. If only I could find the means to expose the reality of what I see—the basal ganglia is like that rowboat, ferrying the mind back and forth between what it can touch and what it can articulate.

—

Like Stanley Fish's "kinetic art," the human body and mind, even in repose, are hardly static. The body and mind respond and shape themselves against the environment, experience, and genetic possibility.

Of course, Robert's disabilities are not "fixed," but endlessly "kinetic," must always be "read" in context, and are constantly shifting, as though Jacques Derrida had produced a piece of living performative theory: my child as a text embodied, perpetually deconstructing and reassembling itself.

In *Self-Consuming Artifacts*, in which Fish breeds reader response theory with Derridean deconstruction, a book whose primary essays I can never finish because the appendix "Literature in the Reader" is so much more interesting, he talks about literature as a kinetic art:

> *The great merit . . . of kinetic art is that it forces you to be aware of "it" as a changing object—and therefore no "object" at all—and also to be aware of yourself as correspondingly changing. Kinetic art does not lend itself to a static interpretation because it refuses to stay still and doesn't let you stay still either. In its operation it makes inescapable the actualizing role of the observer. Literature is a kinetic art, but the physical form it assumes prevents us from seeing its essential nature, even though we so experience it.*

I've been spiritually bound to this quotation since graduate school. It underlies, underlines what I try to do as a poet: make something that has energy and motion, that doesn't revolve, static, on a single, extractable meaning, something that can be entered and exited at a different place each time. Literature as motion, as energy, as the action of the mind across the body of the text.

—

On the other side of this, I am unbearably close and intertwined with Robert on an emotional level. I know what he thinks, I interpret him to the rest of the world, I write him, as it were, upon the psyches of other people. Others gradually take my lead and start to write his person for themselves.

This is how he becomes independent, as much as he can be independent: I take the lead. But adolescence is the time when he should start to take the lead. And I'm not sure how he's going to do that. The kid's a piece of postmodern poetry: most readers aren't willing to leap the gaps, accept the white space as meaningful, wander thoughtfully amid the disjunctures.

I am convinced that "handsome" is a language, though, in and of itself. It's served him well his entire life because people continue to be drawn to him.

—

Disjuncture makes emotional sense to me: that life is a set of fragments, pulled together by sheer will or by semi-passive gathering. Robert is a collection of actions, motivations, and disconnections: a real person who can't speak or act for himself, yet he does "act" and "speak." There are times at which the disjunctures, the re-routings of postmodernism feel viscerally like disability—of circuitous routes toward a goal, circling around a building or winding through the metro looking for a ramp or other means of access. And the relief I feel on finding the accessible entrance to the building is often short-lived as I contemplate the next set of barriers within.

What should make sense, but doesn't: steps, the logical upward platonic ascent toward semantic nirvana—the ladder, the stairs, the single direction all so very static, unimaginative.

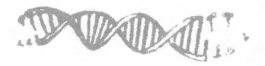

And So Love Any Thing

first born the boy was beautiful
symmetrical in face and limbs body
perfect mechanism people stopped

admired liveliness and smile the way
his hands opened grasped legs kicked
and when he moved he moved more

ways than one *the shapes a bright
container can contain* they'd say or
some such of choice virtues but

then his mechanism broke quite
suddenly stalled stopped restarted
only to fail entirely as vehicles can do

parts in disrepair or in electronic
spark and shudder mutter of some
coding glitch the boy became a

thing word nonspecific for whatever
ceases function although his several
parts kept a pure repose despite

all that he was a martyr to a motion
not his own and still I knew him
lovely in his bones yes he taught me

touch love's tender tenor skin to skin
wiring human hand to hand or face
electric leap offering grace although

surely love must be a thing because
I ask *what thing is love?* my heart's tic toc
this synaptic shock: recognition

Death Valley, California

close to the Nevada border salt
flats dry beds octagonal or hexed

one constant the wind another
dryness the two wicked all away

as though beauty's opposite were
nonconformity absence *things which*

are not what we expected our first
anniversary to be a tour extreme

from desert floor sand-sculpted
to a freezing overlook thousands

of feet high the dusty altitude
blurring distant Proving Grounds

particles like stars seeded thickly
in the deep desert night where I

was afraid unable to connect any
known constellation from so many

stars blinking bright or faint near
or far a cacophony expanding

away from human sight toward
a point of origin *I am life maker*

of worlds as glint scattered by
a neutron star whose compact

darkness births nothing more yet
draws close all *a quintessence even*

from nothingness a not-yet mother
calling softly to an as-yet child

In which I am envious of the Eternal

The valley was full of bones
graves slit to release stillborn stones

of mothers and grandmothers

bones with bracelets of hair
released from sunken faces
of the dying

They stood at his command
the rumble and clack of these
thousand and under them ten thousand more

———————

The Eternal was upon the room
a heavy cloth hanging
we waited for knotted fibers to drop

would he be as he was on the third day?
would we be as we were on the next?

how I had made flesh my own children
how I dressed them with lungs and entrails
how I gently covered their raw bones with
the clean snap of skin, yet

I could not put breath back

(after Ezekiel 37)

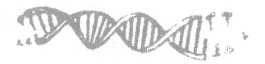

Oscillation

We were all climbing slowly out of a flu-induced fog, through a long weekend of rain oscillating heavy and light against the peaks and valleys of the rooflines, the skylights, and against the black asphalt of the quiet neighborhood street beneath my bedroom window.

When I couldn't quite sleep and couldn't quite rouse myself, my thoughts moved on the road through the valley of the last decade: the tests, drugs, complications. With each failed attempt at diagnosis, another light changed from green to red with barely a flash of yellow in between.

The brakes always went on hard. And, as it happens with life at a certain speed, our habits of thinking, immutable as objects, continued traveling at speed, freed temporarily from reality, until, one by one, they lost velocity and stopped or crashed, as the case might be.

The bumper of a car absorbs impact, bends or creases, gives with the incoming shock, and what doesn't sink in reverberates through the frame and passengers.

While I lay in bed sick, I wondered if that's how an emotional shock works. An event arrives at a certain speed—sometimes you face it, sometimes you look away—and it impacts the soft and hard matter of your body, your self. The way you see things. Such as how I might come to understand whether Robert was constituted of his condition or not and whether the world might come to accommodate him.

Other people see the way an event strikes, but they don't see the shock reverberating through your frame. Because the impact has to go somewhere. It has to dissipate. And sometimes it takes a long time for that shock to travel through your psyche, animating different parts, and where it exits may surprise even you. And it may exit in many places over time.

I lay there thinking that I was never sure if I were moving or standing still. Moving under my own power, or moving with a forward momentum over which I had no control. Standing still as in still standing, or merely stopped.

I remember my favorite few miles of road in the state where I spent so many years of my life—a road I've driven often under different conditions (environmental and emotional) and in different seasons. Its blacktop descends sharply from an open plateau, broad meadows, through a forest and along a creek at the right. On the left are steep banks—a mountain wall.

My memories of this road cast it mostly in dark and shadow, partly because the forest is quite thick, and partly because I've driven the road at night many times—once at three or four in the morning after one of the most significant realizations of my life.

Route 125 is steeply curved and sharply banked. One moment momentum draws the car hard to the right, toward the creek, and then the car is drawn rapidly back toward the mountainside. And again and again. In the dark, headlights catch the sharpest point of each curve, a series of harrowing hairpin shifts, illuminating whatever natural object could have been my demise, before shifting back toward the road and relative safety.

In the dark of my college years, I drove by watching the white line that marks the road's edge, not the center double yellow. And braking judiciously, but not continuously. At that point in my life, such driving could be fun in its own way.

Let's just say I drove this road at intervals during a period when danger of all kinds seemed inviting rather than frightening. But I always felt a twinge of relief the moment the route straightened and leveled and poured itself into the village at the base of the mountain.

The road oscillated between the poles of what could still happen and what hadn't, its energy fading in a village of frame houses that never seemed to change.

Notes on Creativity & Originality

My husband and I set out to have a child in the usual way. Our zygote was, of course, an aspect of our imagination—a he or a she, hair dark or light, eyes bright—we envisioned the future and it was luminous with happiness. We didn't give much thought to the machinations of DNA during our procreative abandonment. We were "making" a baby, which is and isn't like making art. Something was being created beyond our control. We had only imagination to guide us—art's cognitive origin.

Opposite sexes, like my husband and myself, are said to attract and reproduce in a heterogeneous biological pattern (difference), but patterning in art comes from homogeneity, the recognition of likeness, sameness, "giving form," as Mary Shelley wrote in the 1831 preface to *Frankenstein*, to "dark, shapeless substances" and bringing equanimity from disorder, pattern from diversity.

So genetic recombination (the secret of life) might be art's antithesis: two DNA molecules unzip their double strands, nucleic acids release and then join hands with a new partner—a patterning—but each half-strand's original material and biochemical variations rearrange, randomly, to make a blueprint—functional or not—for an organism. Each conception offers a species a potential new direction or a dead end.

Evolution begins with DNA, but Darwin didn't know that. Still, his 1859 theory from *On the Origin of Species* is predicated on chance and happenstance. Species survive crushing environmental blows due to changes in phenotype among certain individuals, which propagate and thrive. Darwin eventually gives in to a temptation to agree with the industrialists and imperialists of his era: evolution serves the purpose of perfecting a species, survival of the fittest.

And yet, modern genetics will prove the social Darwinists wrong. Shifting phenotypes are due to minute glitches in the genome, genetic accidents. Evolution, therefore, might be an opportunistic engine expending energy in multiple directions simultaneously—*not* a progress toward perfection, if that's what art is—or the making of it—revision ever onward toward an ideal. Origin itself points backward toward a source, while artistic originality has connotations of the fresh and new—a drive forward. How to reconcile these root significances, if at all?

By now I know a number of scientists. Recently, one confirmed my belief that the purpose of DNA, or the genome, is to create variation, the unexpected. These random changes to genes during recombination are called "point mutations," which may be of no use to the organism, but any of which might hold the key to species survival down the biological road. Or not. My individual genome is filled with mis-sense, salted with point mutations—everyone has them. Human beings might be the art of chaos.

Although I can't revise him, I go on saying I "made" my son within my body as if I alone created him (without my husband), formed his bones and organs, nurtured his neural connections with the food I ate and the substances I avoided. After all, I considered myself responsible for him.

When he was born, he seemed perfectly normal, indeed beautiful. Just after his first birthday, something broke down abruptly—over mere days. His body has become deformed and distorted; he sometimes drools. I still love him. Always.

David Foster Wallace referred to *Infinite Jest*, his novel-in-progress, as *a kind of hideously damaged infant that follows the writer around ... hydrocephalic and noseless and flipper-armed and incontinent and retarded and dribbling cerebro-spinal fluid out of its mouth as it mewls and blurbles and cries out to the writer, wanting love.* Wallace meant to convey the struggle of writing, the tremendous scope of reconciling ideal and actual, and how it can go so awfully wrong—a creative process gone awry.

A disabled child is certainly an original—what an artist wants?—but in Wallace's conceit, the book-child represents damage, irreparable difference, a failure of creativity.

Of her creative process, Shelley writes, *Invention does not consist in creating out of void, but out of chaos; the materials must, in the first place, be afforded: it can give form to dark, shapeless substances, but cannot bring into being the substance itself.* Untangling this passage requires returning, if not to the absolute origin of certain words, to their knobbly reach into 19th century soil.

By "void," Shelley means "nothing, emptiness." On the other hand, her "chaos" contains the unidentifiable precursors of beings, things, ideas. Kind of like fetal cells rapidly dividing from two to eight to sixteen to hundreds and thousands, then specializing into cell types, which become nerve and muscle and bone tissue.

Shelley, though, isn't talking life, she's discussing literary creation. "Invention" was that process that gave "form to dark, shapeless substances," and for two hundred years it had several stages, the first of which was "imitatio," or finding a well-known concept or image from which a writer might develop her own ingenious variation—creativity as collaboration between artist and culture, creativity as (re)production, not originality as we understand it. By Shelley's time, a terrifically good "invention" was beginning to imply artistic "genius" (from "ingenium")—to make something *original* or new from the void of the self's deep well, like gods, not parents.

Or perhaps she's discussing more than literary creation. For generations before her time, when biological reproduction was discussed, men were said to provide the "homunculus" (fetus) with "form," while women provided "matter" or "substance." When she says that invention *can give form to dark, shapeless substances, but cannot bring into being the substance itself,* she's mingling tropes about both human and literary creativity. She has to. She's a woman writing fiction.

"Chaos," is the female principle of creation, its womb, that from which arises substance—if, and only if, given "form," by a masculine principle. In the psychology of that era, the imagination was a womb-like part of the brain from which ideas could be drawn for refinement by higher thought processes such as reason and judgment. By arguing that invention itself gives form, and suggesting all writers may possess a capacity for invention, she argues that writing (art) itself is hermaphroditic, not exclusively a male prerogative.

But, and this "but" has significance for her peers: if art is reproduction apart from some "natural" law of creation (say, that of a Judeo-Christian god), is genius unnatural? What are the consequences and license of true artistic originality?

All the above terms exist uncomfortably in the full text of her 1831 preface, mixing and remixing: Can there be true creative originality? Or is originality a dangerous hubris? This uneasiness infiltrates the novel: Victor Frankenstein, the monster's creator, "invents" by piecing together stolen corpses in the hope of manifesting his genius to the world—he believes he's discovered the secret of life. He believes he can create something original, like a god. *I became myself capable of bestowing animation upon lifeless matter.*

Frankenstein can be read not only as a warning about the dangers of science, but as a cautionary tale of the artist's hubris, let alone the responsibility of an artist or parent to her creation. Consider our hubris: my husband and I created our son thinking he would be a reflection of ourselves, a test of our own creativity. We "made" him. An animate example of our genius.

We spent 14 years trying to understand what had happened to our creation, taking him from one research neurologist to another, testing for this and for that—medical science is always advancing, morphing in different directions as new bits of information become available. When genome sequencing, a test that "reads" all three billion letters of human DNA, moved from research to clinical use, we jumped at it. By now we knew the answer lay somewhere in his genes.

While we were waiting for the sequencing results, a friend asked me, *What does it matter to find a diagnosis, if there's no cure?* I could rewrite this, Why bother with a draft you can't revise?

When scientists converse, "matter" represents physical substance: whatever has mass and takes up space. When the rest of us talk, "matter" is most often an emotional state: this matters, that doesn't matter. To say something "doesn't matter," however, suggests it means nothing, which might be the same as saying it doesn't exist— "lifeless matter." Can my son not matter to anyone, yet still have mass and take up space?

Frankenstein was inspired not only by a ghost story competition, but by the philosophical talk among Shelley's set that summer of 1816: *the nature of the principle of life, and whether there was any probability of its ever being discovered and communicated.* Shelley reported the question most asked of her since the novel's 1818 publication had been, "How I, then a young girl, came to think of and to dilate upon so very hideous an idea?" The cervix dilates during childbirth, opening and expanding.

Her novel is framed as a seaman's tale, elaborately nested within multiple narrations. It dilates from the center: the abandoned monster tells his story to Victor; Victor tells that and his own story to Robert Walton (an aspiring scientist who has rescued Victor); Walton writes it down in a letter he sends to his sister.

At the center, the monster wonders whether his evil results from his original nature (dead bodies) or nurture (Victor's abandonment)— Shelley's "hideous idea" embedded as an unresolved question about human nature, creativity and art that David Foster Wallace will echo 150 years later: *The fiction always comes out so horrifically defective … a cruel and repellent caricature of the perfection of its conception - yes, understand: grotesque because imperfect. And yet it's yours, the infant is, it's you, and you love it.* Of course.

Amid these intimations, one might form analogies among human creativity, artistic creativity and scientific knowledge:

- Originality: whatever the imagination conceives first appears deformed, defective.
- Creativity: a labor of love to perfect the imperfect.
- Biological origin: DNA.
- Biological creation: the application of energy to matter, such that the resulting organism grows and breathes; gestation.

Originality : creativity :: defective : perfect;

originality : creativity :: DNA : gestation;

DNA : imperfect :: gestation : perfect;

DNA : lovemaking :: imagination : creative energy; or

DNA : creative energy :: lovemaking : imagination.

In February 1953, Francis Crick burst into a Cambridge pub shouting, *We have discovered the secret of life!*, much to the dismay of James Watson, who worried the announcement was premature. Nevertheless, in April of 1953, *Nature* published Watson and Crick's Nobel Prize-winning paper, "A Structure for Deoxyribose Nucleic Acid."

Scientific work never occurs in a void; it arises from the chaos of competition. *Nature* published several articles in its April issue under the heading, "Molecular Structure of Nucleic Acids," including papers by Watson and Crick's competitors: Franklin and Gosling; Wilkins, Stokes and Wilson. Each of these scientists, along with many who came before, contributed to the big discovery: DNA. Centuries of wonder reached a pinnacle with Watson and Crick's proof that the helix is doubled and the phosphates are on the outside, capable of reproducing per the laws of molecular chemistry.

The origin of a story or of life might be a chain of linked phosphates swirling around the recombinant vortex into which an artist's creativity sinks and then rises. White phosphorus glows upon exposure to oxygen, breathing the first necessary act of any newly created organism. Oxidative phosphorylation is the chemical name for the cellular respiratory chain, the body's primary source of energy. *As if to breathe were life!*, Tennyson has Ulysses complain. In fact, it is.

At the cellular level *we return to a plain sense of things*, the end of the creative imagination borne out as chemicals, *inanimate in an inert savoir*, or so goes Wallace Stevens" poem, "The Plain Sense of Things." Stevens wrote most of the poems in *The Rock* (1954) during the late 1940s and early 1950s, at the height of the race to identify DNA. The poem's first lines are:

> *After the leaves have fallen, we return*
> *To a plain sense of things. It is as if*
> *We had come to an end of the imagination,*
> *Inanimate in an inert savoir.*

The phrase "the end of the imagination" comes first, and then Stevens writes, "the *absence* of the imagination had itself to be imagined." All this an odd leap of metaphysics: the admission of an end of creativity, and then the suggestion of a void—as though the answer to our existence were a secret only gods or scientists might know, something that precedes the animate, some inorganic principle that could give form to lifeless matter.

"Inanimate in an inert savoir": French distinguishes between *savoir*, to know absolutely, and *connaître*, to understand through familiarity and suggestion. Within the spelling of these hide shadows of other verbs: *voir*, to see, and *naître*, to be born, as though one can know absolutely only what can be seen with the eyes, and as though true understanding might be as intimate as birth, female bodily creativity.

What we know absolutely we know not through any *ordinary* human creativity. Watson, Crick, Franklin, Wilkins and the rest were obsessed with knowledge absolute. Not with what matters, but with what can be seen, observed, proven.

The first time I read *Moby Dick*, the professor handed us "The Plain Sense of Things," to mull in relation to the ruinous glory of Ahab's obsession.

A bit like Ahab, my husband and I persisted through years of testing, certain one day absolute data would explain our child's disabilities. For years, the tests came back negative or normal: with each result we were released from our worst imaginings, the worst diagnoses. We lived in the eddy of each end, and, then, each absence. *The absence of the imagination had itself to be imagined.* I visualized diagnosis as a whale emerging from the sea, too big to be seen all at once—the back, the tail, the tips of the flukes, the blow-hole, the crest of the head—each of these parts surfacing and slip-sliding away back into the sea before my mind had a fix on the glimpse.

The truth, though, was very small. Three billion nucleotides compose a single strand of DNA. On one of his chromosome 2 copies, our son inherited a point mutation from me on the PRKRA gene—a defect so rare it had been reported in the medical literature only 8 times. On the other, from my husband, there is a *de novo* defect on PRKRA—one nucleotide switched out for another, but a different point mutation than the variant I gave him. In genetics, "de novo" means "new; never before seen." Entirely original. Most likely, our geneticist said, the *de novo* variant was the result of a gamete transcription error by my husband's RNA, and that spermatozoa just happened to unite with my ovum. A one in three billion chance happening.

There was no answer to the question of which of us had been responsible for our child's illness. The chaos of my body had carried this unexpressed defect forward through many generations. My husband didn't carry the defect he'd given our son. In the relatively ordered world of gamete production, a simple typo had been made. Some typos are barely noticeable and do not affect a reader's relationship with a text. Others create unidentifiable words that affect the intent of a sentence, a paragraph, a novel. What did Shelley really mean? Or Wallace?

Genome sequencing analyzes the biochemical building blocks of each gene: adenine, cytosine, guanine, thymine, or ACGT. All life is composed by a four-letter alphabet spelling out 23,000 active genes. Interruptions in the patterns of ACGT may cause a shift, small or large, malignant or benign, in the regulation of biochemical processes.

One analogy is with a computer: underneath programs (body functions), an operating system (DNA, or the genome)—under that, binary computer code composed of the numerals 1 and 0 (nucleotides) arranged in infinitely complex patterns, that make sense and function, unless a programmer skips a 1 or inserts an extra 0.

And that is, perhaps, David Foster Wallace's anxiety: *The fiction always comes out so horrifically defective ... a cruel and repellent caricature of the perfection of its conception.* He might become that errant programmer—the anxiety of revision reflected in every comma placement, a need for each word to be precise. Yet, does Wallace follow in Darwin's errant footsteps? Must the evolution of the text result in the perfection of the genre?

Shelley might be said to argue female writers have an advantage — the imagination like a chaotic womb, realization and discovery dilating like a cervix. We have the right parts to fully know creativity on the street or in the boudoir.

Wallace might long for an hermaphroditism he worries he might lack: *even at the height of its hideousness the damaged infant somehow touches and awakens what you suspect are some of the very best parts of you: maternal parts, dark ones. You love your infant very much. And you want others to love it, too.*

Early modern numerology makes much of the resemblance of 1 and 0 to male and female genitalia, one and nothing, or "no thing," which might be why computer coding and the approach of artificial intelligence have people so concerned. The secret of consciousness could be long white strands of just those two numerals, numinous against the glow of a blue or black screen. Digital sex, stripped of emotion and attachment.

At the end of *Moby Dick*, as the womb of the sea closes on the sinking ship, the final twirl of the vortex spits out a coffin, on which Ishmael floats to safety, to the ship *Rachel*, "in her retracing search after her missing children." The ocean's spiral makes a zero and the coffin shapes a one, a metaphysical reproduction undone and re-done in the wake of Ishmael's survival. Sometimes I think of DNA's double-helix as a 3-D dilation, a vortex opening the very language of life, a variant of art, some type of creativity beyond human intellectual capacity.

Discovering the structure of DNA meant only that scientists knew which chemical components of a cell were responsible for genetic replication. The "secret of life" can come only when we understand how each gene of DNA is encoded or wrongly coded. Then we can "read" our own history and individual life stories. We know our son's PRKRA gene encodes erroneous proteins, but we do not yet understand how these errant proteins provoke cellular chaos. We cannot stop it, nor can we revise his gene, although that day may come. Still, we persist. As David Foster Wallace said, *You love your infant very much. And you want others to love it, too.*

Or Shelley, *I bid my hideous progeny go forth and prosper. I have an affection for it, for it was the product of happy days.* Love matters.

We fear difference: dis-abling breaks in an evolving human pattern that cannot be revised or resolved. At the same time we think we love flesh and blood, whatever is "human," and fear the polished ultra-perfection of artificial intelligence. We contradict ourselves—we are large, we contain multitudes (ah, Whitman, father of American literature).

One and zero, something and nothing, four nucleotides, twenty-six letters. Three of us—Shelley, Wallace, myself—with our "hideous" texts. In the various languages of creativity and originality, it would seem my son is doomed forever. He cannot be revised or repaired—his creation a matter of happenstance and chaos. Yet he grows and breathes, has mass and takes up space—*de novo*, he's entirely original, without precedence or pattern.

Pattern: if that's what art is. Originality: whatever breaks or confounds established patterns to create new templates; genius. Does Stevens suggest his greatness is such that art ends with him, *inanimate in an inert savoir?*

Perhaps more frightening, do these terms—creativity, originality, genius, pattern, matter—reach consensus only when what links them is beauty, or human perfection? Because it seems beauty, that most time-worn pattern of all, can never be original—only the hideous can meet that criteria. *You want to sort of fool people,* wrote Wallace, *You want them to see as perfect what you in your heart know is a betrayal of all perfection.*

If DNA in its energetic and variant-prone replication represents the secret of life, and art is life distilled, are beauty and perfection truly the essence of art? I hope not. What matters in art, life, science, must be attendant to both pattern and disruption. Shelley wrote, *Invention consists in the capacity of seizing on the capabilities of a subject: and in the power of moulding and fashioning ideas suggested to it.*

What matters is human chaos, imagination's womb, the point mutation of originality. Matter cannot be revised or perfected, it simply exists, having mass and taking up space—but its properties and aspect can be seized upon and transformed by creative energy into whatever we are willing to love and accept as art—or humanity. If we insist upon perfection, the imagination may end with inertia, in the hubris of Stevens" inanimate void.

Disability & Space-Time Considerations

One Boy. I thought of that while walking home from dropping Robert at his inclusive theater class. The sun was shining, construction ongoing, tall buildings sending steel beams into the sky. I'd read a book on quantum physics while drinking my morning coffee. Something about imagining the scale of atomic parts. Something about the nucleus of an atom being like a grain of sand inside a 14-story building, the building itself mostly empty, a handful of electrons—smaller still than sand—whirring from floor to floor.

Then there's the subatomic. At that level, Newtonian physics ceases to apply, yet patterns can accrue. Or not. And buildings still may stand, erected on a sort of quantum shifting sand invisible to the naked eye.

As electrons jump from orbit to orbit, shell to shell of an atom, excited and turned on by whatever energy is applied to them, we can't see them. Yet these particles leave traces of themselves ("light fingerprints") in the wavelengths of light around us. These can be measured by spectrography, but we can't know which electrons will jump to which shell of the atom or why, only measure the probability of the density of such a gathering of minutia on any given band. We don't so much *know* as *calculate* the probability of knowing—that's the initial understanding I have of how quantum physics imagines a world, all within the estimable boundaries of mathematics as a form of language rather than a measure of absolute knowledge.

That the boundaries of science might be permeable after all, elastic, without absolutes gives me hope. Everything is relative! from Aristotle's teachings on rhetoric to particle physics. Because if the world really were absolute, then One Boy wouldn't matter.

And I mean that literally—as an anomaly, he would have no matter, no substance, nothing to him would accrue. He'd have no value; interest accrues to investments, for example. The financial world thrives on absolutes: winners and losers, spread sheets, bottom lines. Science may be relative, but money may be a god, despite the disclaimer on our currency, *In god we trust*. Gods, some think, should be absolute. And yet, the gold standard is no more. Even finance these days is speculative, derivative, incomprehensible, and, ultimately, collapsible.

Peter Higgs first theorized the Higgs bosun, the "god particle," in 1964, the year I was born. This subatomic particle, elusive, invisible, lacking quantitative measurements to prove its existence, marks the point at which matter, well, matters. Some theoretical physicists describe it as a celebrity moving through a crowd, gathering admirers—gaining mass, taking up space. The scientific definition of "matter."

The Higgs bosun only makes itself known to us as it emerges from destruction (literally), and from there, the world we know may be assembled as atoms, molecules, deoxyribose nucleic acid, cells, bacteria, eukaryotes, multicellular organisms. Molecules, elements, electronic forces, hammers, screws, machines, buildings.

Still, One Boy has an uneasy glow. Why does one person matter? One person with as unique a biochemical profile as anyone might imagine. Or not. Robert is, of course, more like any of us than he is different. Only two errors among the three billion nucleotides of his genome. He's still human, after all.

I can't explain why one person matters. I don't know that an explanation exists. The quanta in quantum physics simply assume that a measurement for the unknown and undefinable exists. In one version of the universe, for every bit of matter, there's an equal and opposite bit of anti-matter, dark matter. As One Boy moves through space-time, how do the particles of society react to him, how does he gather support? From the draw of recognition (a positive charge) or the simultaneous push and pull of a negative charge, a distancing empathy?

Physicists push and pull over two theories of the universe: Super Symmetry or the Multiverse. The familiar harmony of the poets sings forth in Super Symmetry, a world in which all things are balanced, ordered, and beautiful. The Multiverse posits innumerable parallel universes, each with its own laws of physics—disorder, chaos, in which beauty implodes into particles of randomness.

In a sprawling universe, say the Multiverse proponents, our galaxy, even our entire universe, is just one among many, each beginning perhaps with a separate bang and expansion. If worlds do collide, will their inhabitants be intelligible one to the other?

I've been raised to believe in beauty, symmetry and order, yet the inexplicable appeals to me, too. Says one famous physicist, *The idea of the multiverse would move us to a real picture, not of symmetry and beauty and order, but fundamentally of chaos on enormous distances.*

The Higgs bosun matters *because* it is unstable—the point of destruction at which all matter accrues, Higgs gives its being so that other particles may have mass. A messiah? Perhaps Lord Shiva instead. A creator and destroyer all-in-one, so the theory goes, this "god" particle might become visible only when speed and force recreate conditions of the Big Bang.

And so the Large Hadron Collider was constructed over ten years, from 1998 (the year Robert became disabled) to 2008. In 2012, the year Robert was diagnosed, the LHC proved the existence of the Higgs bosun. The numerical value of the Higgs, physicists hoped, would prove the universe conformed to the laws of Super Symmetry, or rebelled in the form of a Multiverse.

Its only measurements mathematical—waves and points and digits—thus far, the Higgs numerical value sits, taunting, in between symmetry and chaos.

The Higgs bosun only appears at the point at which other matter destructs. The LHC can run the experiment over and over again, pattern-upon-pattern accruing data, the method of understanding a universe caught between repetition and the unexpected.

If the parts of an atom have a scale like that of a 14-story building, and the atoms of a baseball would, to scale, take up the mass of the world, how do we find each other, attract one another, create other human beings in mutual accordance, parse the parameters and direction of motion and intent across the inconceivable volume of space-time? Let alone find answers to the questions that perplex us?

Let there be anomalies within anomalies, as long as we may find something to know. For every theory there's an outlier, something that cannot be predicted or understood. What drives financiers and economists? Gain, value, a hoped for symmetry of economic return.

What drives art? Discovery of pattern among randomness, inconsistency, or, I hope, an acceptance of inconsistency. Is it too simple to hope the art of outliers may be recognition and connection, rather than acceptance of typical human pattern? In any symmetrical system, can One Boy be anything more than negligible? Or could a multiverse contain all of us, each and every One?

Pure science offers no thought of gain or reward, says another physicist, *The things that are least important for our survival are the very things that make us human.* He's a believer in Super Symmetry.

We don't see answers; we can't. Only know that particles leave traces in wavelengths of light as electrons jump from shell to shell, excited only because energy has been applied to them—the electrons don't know why. Measure the density on any given band; calculate the probability of knowing. Mass can accrue from the instability of what surrounds it—in fact, is brought into being by fracture and chaos, symmetry and order. Antithesis. Antimatter. One Boy.

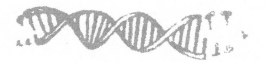

Life as We Know It

Best left to physicists' eyes sharpened finer than nanometers:
atoms, particles, quantum leaps where materiality recedes

so that proportionate space though small may be infinite as
star distance marked by fusion clusters, the hydro-helium

macrocosm where our sun alight gives leave to plants' silent
respiration in turn to us recidivists who breathe, our DNA

from comets, inorganic pyrimidine bases, angles symmetric
build us up like all the world from elements, blur of electrons

subatomic distances throughout which light still is constant
where being slings along the warp and weft of space-time,

relativity, to parse a world *whose margin fades forever when we move*
beyond empiric and yet we rest organic, measurable: nucleo-

tides tracing glassine curls the double helix with its ramrod
stairs, forms microcosmic or shades of cyto-stains blue red

or green, ACGT these four fates spell select or forfeit, spin
and cut unseen: destiny or chance mutation? *de novo* variant

will write a newer world, new chance at (r)evolution, our
oulipo novel a workshop of potential, no plot to form or

character to find *that which we are, we are* words entangled
in a nucleus, cell empire amidst chatter genetic, busy capitol:

around float organelles, mitochondria cytoplasmic galleons,
within row transport chains, electrons that cannot rest from

travel (oxidative phosphorylation): neg pos neg pos neg
(pause) complete circuit, a redox reaction in eternal redux

as though to breathe were life indeed, its generator, oxygen's power sputters and that energy drives bodily fission and fusion

until death when we return to form *a part of all that we have
met:* elements, atoms, the quanta where materiality recedes

into uncertainty disorder and revision, particles super- or
sub- atomic, where little remains yet large in eternal redux

Meiosis

soft bellies of infants come to mind
     all unprotected flesh rounded to touch
smell of their fine hair like cilia prompts
     uterine clench, staunch of breath *obstinate*
questionings of sense and outward things
     a maker central centromere, an X that
forms as chromosomes double and
     thicken: a mutagenic sea unseen *nothing*
can bring back the hour now drowsy
     with creative energy we look down from
high cliffs while shearing gusts
     ripple a surface nosing the shore falling
back, fading to what floats beyond
     the surf, *birth is but a sleep and a forgetting*
while ribonucleic acid makes its way
     a clipper rolling with the swell, parting
double strands of whatever may
     happen or come to being, to replicate
the moment, a linguistic intention
     letters ACGT have no primal sympathy
no patience for endless imitation as if
     their whole vocation were to repeat not
quite those things that had been said
     before as this messenger along a frozen
sea of beauty in division, snips parent
     from parent prepares for recombination
some fragment a hastening or quickening
     from a dream of human life not yet precise
in the telling rigging chance poetics
     as sailors might rounding Cape Horn lashed
to the mast unprotected flesh braced
     for the moment somatic seas clash, stipple
of salt water splendor before nucleo-
     tides swell and recede, attach disentangle
genetic ropes and leads, chromosomes
     fading to fetal strands, curling invisible
for now intimations, tangles of heredity

After Life

I asked my mother
where they went
in the dark a closed door
child's step on tile
no one spoke not even she

we dreamed on the docks
night lake a glass plate
far edge set a line of solder
at the horizon blue black
before the stars emerged

and it slid back at us
overheard adult voices
cathartic laughter echoing
they went into love the inky
dim and infinite scatter

gravel spotting the water
surface irregular something
before sinking that's what
she might have told me
had I wanted to know

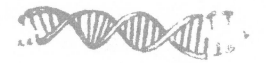

Tomb of the Unknown

I want to find more answers, but I don't know how. Maybe that's how love is.

Or maybe not. Love seemed the least of it sometimes. Order was all my husband and I had asked for—to look into Robert's genome after fourteen years of medical review without answers, into the human echo, winding double rails of a spiral stairwell, "helix" in geometry, to understand what might be the displacement among three billion genetic letters in this unknown disease.

Perhaps our energy and faith had become a mathematics of devotion. I could count for you the number of biopsies, surgeries, blood tests, genetic tests. How many medications we tried to help him regain some movement. Our interventions were all about helping his quality of life, I swear.

After thirteen years of waiting for the medical future to arrive, we were offered genomic sequencing. Space-age, engine of time, a computer would read his molecules of DNA and encode each one—adenine, thymine, guanine, cytosine—as letters, ACGT. If it were a library, human DNA would fill one million pages, or make four thousand average-length books.

There are 3 billion nucleotides on each strand of human DNA. So many nucleotides form a gene, so many genes dot a chromosome, and we all have two chromosomes to prevent genetic disaster, or at least stave it off. On each of his chromosome 2 copies, Robert has variants, defects, mutations (choose whichever word you please) to the PRKRA gene, implicated in muscle function.

We know now what is out of step, can ascribe numerals to it—point mutations c.665C>T and c.637T>C—but we cannot change or alter it.

At Arlington National Cemetery, along the wall of a sweeping granite plaza next to the Eternal Flame are inscribed a cluster of quotations from JFK's sole inaugural address, including this effort at prophesy:

The Energy - the Faith - the Devotion
Which we bring to this endeavor
Will light our country
And all who serve it
And the glow from that fire
Can truly light the world

I visit Arlington regularly, mostly for the view from the Custis-Lee Mansion on the promontory above the river, from which I can see the entire city of Washington DC receding into the distance on the far shore of the Potomac.

The precise rows of graves with uniform headstones align and realign themselves, moving within peripheral vision as I walk by: the last resting spot for some 400,000 soldiers, politicians, and dignitaries. Each small white stone forms a mark on green grass, so many feet or inches separated from the one to its left, right, front, back.

If you go to Arlington, the graves undulating over 624 acres will seem an immense, unimaginable number, and your throat may constrict as you consider the toll of war. That would be an understandable human reaction.

We think of the genome as precise, as precise as the changing of the guard at the Tomb of the Unknown. A lone patrol strides with an exacting heel-to-foot roll along a red carpet for 21 steps, turns and faces the tomb for 21 seconds, and reverses direction.

Changing the guard brings forward two more soldiers, the relief commander and the relief sentinel. The two honor guards march in parallel while the commander joins, inspects and separates them—a tempting analogy to the role of RNA in DNA replication.

But the mathematics of devotion the U.S. Armed Forces can bring to any task may be far more precise than the body. In the military, chain of command is absolute. Among our cells and their marching orders, not so much.

Disease resulting from errors to PRKRA is called dystonia 16, a gradually progressive illness, of which Robert is the ninth reported case in the world, the first in the U.S. Because of his *de novo* variant, his symptoms are worse than any of the other eight reported cases.

Of those eight I know nothing except one liners: a consanguineous family in Brazil, a person of indeterminate age in Germany who has, also, a heterozygous recessive case, but not a *de novo* defect.

I've always been afraid of the number nine. Not because Sesame Street gave me nightmares, but because near the end of high school, I picked up a book in the library on numerology. I can't recall the title, although in my memory the book's cover is always black.

I stood with my shoulder against the bookshelf, those grey metal industrial rows, leafing through it. One chapter promised it held the key to fate through the addition of the numerical value of names and birthdates. My numerical fate turned out to be nine, which, the book informed me, was the worst possible number: I would always come very close to achieving something, but never make it. My life would be a pattern of incompleteness.

So I shut the cover.

If I'd never opened the cover, never read the chapter, would the numerical value of my identity have been a silent secret metaphysical presence throughout my days?

The point is, Robert's genomic variants were there all along, from the moment of his conception to the moment of his neuromuscular unravelling to the moment of their discovery—small prophetic messages as mundane as the daily lives of the native inhabitants of the Americas until Columbus landed and claimed their very ordinary in the name of Spanish sovereigns.

At the Eternal Flame, some visitors weep. The story of the Kennedy family is a tragic one: two children assassinated, one killed at war, another in a plane crash, one had a developmental disorder, and the rest are gradually aging or dying of terrible diseases. JFK and RFK's assassinations still breed conspiracy theories and proto-myths, as though this family's constellation of suffering has an origin in the prophetic and not mere accidents of existence accrued unfairly.

I cried, too, after the origin of Robert's illness became known to us. One night, a couple of weeks into this new order of things, I woke in a state of shock—maybe I'd been dreaming, maybe I hadn't—and in an awful cliché not my entire life, but images and snippets of the last 14 years were flashing through my mind and I couldn't make them stop—Robert at the table at our old house, now at our new one, images of the school bus, holidays, trips, hospitalizations, all of it. In each image, the disease had marked him in a different way.

That seemed to be the point of the slide show projected on the frontal lobe of my brain: each nexus of his difference connected to every other one. The blue screen on a computer after the device warns you in tight white type that a complete data dump has begun and the bytes scroll by rapid-fire, faster than my brain could read—that's what it was like. Recovery error. I found myself face-down on the carpet, sobbing.

How one reacts to a discovery of that impossibly small magnitude is debatable, one among many explicable human reactions. It's a matter of interpretation. Maybe love can be so strong that the making of a single person from two bends the laws of biochemistry such that like must have like, even to the last detail. Or maybe it's just a coincidence.

The Custis-Lee Mansion, or the land around it, was seized by President Lincoln during the Civil War. General Robert E. Lee was the current owner of the property, and legend has it that Lincoln wanted the war dead buried in Lee's front yard. For the rest of his life, Lee would have to look out over the dead from a war the administration felt he could have prevented. Standing on the portico, I see that, in the distance across the river, the Arlington Memorial Bridge makes a sight line directly to the Lincoln Memorial, as if on purpose, to spite Lee further from the grave. A grudge.

The last time I visited, the tour guide said none of those stories were true.

Inscribed on the Tomb of the Unknown Solider: *Here rests in honored glory an American soldier known but to God.* That, too, has become a fiction. Scientists have read DNA script from the bones of the dead and returned their identities—but not their remains—home.

One of my mother's favorite sayings is "self-fulfilling prophesy." She thinks one can think too much, and has had a concern I go over events too often, looking for a meaning that probably isn't there. But there are times I wonder if I "go over" whatever it is enough, maybe the bad parts will disappear.

I might believe if I over-think things, I may be able to re-invent them. Nine might be the penultimate, the number before the next deca-whatever starts. It may well be making it almost to the pinnacle, yet having to cede that to ten. But it's also a point of waiting, a point of attention, attendance, expectation. The moment before the page flips to, perhaps, an answer. The antechamber of possibility.

We waited 14 years, 1 + 4 = 5, the number of perfect harmony of man and woman, to find our answer, which was a 9. Adding 9 + 14 yields 23, which digits add to 5. Maybe our love might be strong enough yet to learn a new mathematics of devotion.

And yet I will start once more where I began: I want to find more answers, but I don't know how.

Grief

Over the phone, an old friend tells me he has a serious illness. The disease has kept company with him for several years. During the three decades I've known this man, we've often shared secrets, but at other times we don't speak for years. I am opened clean as an abandoned clam shell, silky opalescent interior exposed, edges sharp as a razor.

I know something of grief. When my son fell ill, friends and acquaintances handed me packages of grief as though I would need sadness or know what to do with theirs. I put these bags and parcels in the back of a mental closet, where I stored my true feeling: primal terror. I kept this door closed so my son would not be afraid.

As a child, I often cut my feet on clam shells. The most painful cuts were between the toes; these never seemed to heal, flaps of skin separating bloodlessly months later. Freshwater clams opened on the sandy bottom of Malletts Bay amid the milfoil: dark green wavering, many-branched plants that grow in Lake Champlain. Near the milfoil swam clusters of minnows we'd try to scoop into buckets—water resisted us, and the small fish darted in formation off and away.

My grandfather would curse the invasive milfoil each summer, as its strange beauty choked out other aquatic plants, its line of incursion steadily toward shore. The weed grows so thickly, swimmers become entangled, rudders and motors stall. Like love gone awry, milfoil's feathery tentacles envelop all.

My body gestated my son and daughter's bodies, the food I ate converted to energy for their needs, each presence felt internally first, the quick movements of a fish. Later my husband and I recognized the press of a hand, head or foot through layers of uterine wall, fatty tissue, muscle and epidermis. I have never been closer to anyone than my children. My husband and I can be physically "close," bare skin pressed to the same, yet he can never cross my body's barriers, only knock at the door of my cervix.

Intimacy—emotional or physical—seems at the heart of grief—or rather, the sudden lack of these. Touch eliminates distance, dissolving barriers, whether platonic or sensual. My grief for anyone I have embraced becomes fathomless: fathom from the Old English word for "out-stretched arms," fingertip-to-fingertip the generations of loves go into the murk and deep.

Sex may be the most secret part of love *per* all its forms, but each day streets teem publicly with the products of it. Through a linked chain of bodies, parents and grandparents, I entered the world, an untouchable, intimate taboo.

My grandfather built a summer house into a forested hillside above Malletts Bay when his own children were young. To reach the camp, as we called it, we descended three flights of stairs from our parked car in pine-shade. The building dug in on pilings, cross-beamed, canvas curtains in lieu of doors, living space above, bedrooms below. He built a staircase, now gray with age, more than two stories from the camp to the beach, the last dozen steps emerging from forest twilight into brilliant sun on quartz sand. Why he placed the building so precariously on that steep slope, I can't say, yet it remains firmly planted there 50 years later.

I associate my grandfather, who loved poetry, with Robinson Jeffers. Both were dedicated to untouched wilderness, abhorred cities, treasured their freedom *(live free or die)*. I think of him when I read Jeffers' poem "The Purse-Seine," about sardine fishermen who work at night off the coast of California.

> *I cannot tell you*
> *How beautiful the scene is, and a little terrible, then, when the*
>   *crowded fish*
> *Know they are caught, and wildly beat from one wall to the other*
>   *of their closing destiny the phosphorescent*
> *Water to a pool of flame, each beautiful slender body sheeted with*
>   *flame, like a live rocket*

I feel grief most intensely in these lines: suspended animation of thrashed water, beauty and terror at once, the fish so vividly physical

I can touch the shine of bodies, velvet sting of seawater and rough cords of the net.

Damp hair combed, bodies still dusted with the smell of sand and lake algae, nothing felt better than slipping between my grandmother's cotton sheets, the softest and purest I have ever felt. After lights out, we listened to the distant lap and roll as waves moved on without us into the night, open windows letting in night chill even during July.

One of the largest freshwater lakes in the world, Lake Champlain's shoreline wends its way around the lake edge 587 miles. When I was young, the lake seemed infinite, towns on the opposite shore pinpricks of light at night, the day-time beauty of it a glittering 435 square miles of surface, only a fraction seen from our perch on Malletts Bay. I loved the shore, but rarely ventured by boat into the center—on average 12 persons deep—because I fear death by drowning most.

A mentor says I'll eventually mark time by illnesses and funerals, just as it passes now a knotted string of weddings and birth announcements. Standing in a parking lot after class, metal carapaces in rows, I had just mentioned my surprise watching the memorial service at Ground Zero. A college classmate's age had been announced: 37. For a second, I knew that couldn't be right because I was 38.

At a party, this classmate had kissed me, his lips thick and wet, the two of us in a shadowed corner of his fraternity while drunken people shouted and spilled beer, music blaring. His hips pressed against my body felt awkward and his lips didn't move me. I found a reason to excuse myself.

After the planes and the towers, I learned he had perished. It was none of my business—I had no right to grieve—but I obsessed over knowing where and how he'd died—so much of each company's personnel was written up in the papers. When I realized he might have been one of a group that exited one tower due to fire in the other, then returned to their desks, I became unhinged. The part about returning, unknowing, to danger gets me each time, such a trust in those buildings, that the world's structure would remain inviolate.

A late complication brought us breathlessly to the hospital before our son was born. A technician passed a paddle slick with lubricant across my belly and the boy-to-be appeared, lovely and perfectly formed, so clearly I could almost catch the expression on his fetal face, which flickered between skin and skull. The tech said his image could not quite be captured, his bones not yet dense enough to repel sound waves.

My friend and I talk about his illness, the particulars, the statistics, for over an hour. I am calm, determined not to hand him a satchel filled with my grief. Once we hang up, I can't quite get the words out to my husband. After he gently pulls these out of me, I cry myself to sleep while he curls close to me in bed. I sob on and off all the next day, but I realize, selfishly, that my sadness stems in part from a concern my friend, a support to me through my son's long illness, and whom I thought would always be there, well, maybe he won't. Repeatedly, I shove back a regret that we've never been physically intimate, although I've seen his body undressed. I wonder if grief even qualifies as an emotion, whether it might be a weed that digs its tentacles into the softest matter of my brain.

When I turned, his face was inches from mine, and the abstractions of our attraction collapsed within our lips, teeth, and tongues. We were young then, whatever illnesses that might claim either of us sunk deep in the chthonic, chance iterations of our genomes. My own will surface one day. My friend and I admitted to each other much later that the kiss was a first true intimacy, a safety, and I think this the reason I still cannot let go of him, despite the fact I married another. But now I consider my memories of this kiss self-indulgent, the way a finger traces the opal sheen inside a shell to feel the smoothness, while the dark layers of cuticle and calcium on the outside lay rough against the palm.

The papers reported my classmate's group went toward the roof or the observation deck for rescue. Once, I stood on that observation deck where, the pamphlet said, you could see for 50 miles on a clear day. I remember the city's grid laid out in miniature below me, a sharp breath and my chest tightening as I looked down. Beauty and terror. I am embarrassed to say I could not stay away from even the last detail: in an interview, his wife said their new home on a lake remained half-finished; they'd dreamed of looking out over the water.

Whenever I meditate on loving-kindness, I do as the meditation suggests, expand from myself to those close to me to total strangers, *even all of humankind*, the tape says. I repeat, silently, the key phrases, *may you be safe, may you be free from suffering, may you be healed, may you know peace.* Sometimes I add, *shanti, shanti, shanti,* the Sanskrit knotting me with past, present and future strands of human longing.

In Jeffers' poem, there's no peace, only a refraction of all human terror from a great distance:

> *Lately I was looking from a night mountain-top*
> *On a wide city, the colored splendor, galaxies of light: how could I*
> *help but recall the seine-net*
> *Gathering the luminous fish? I cannot tell you how beautiful the*
> *city appeared, and a little terrible.*
> *I thought, We have geared the machines and locked all together*
> *into interdependence; we have built the great cities; now*
> *There is no escape.*

How beautiful the net of the city shining at night, gathering bodies that trust it to protect and to provide, and yet the poet, sorrowful for the lot of us trapped, calls our attention to his own autonomy, as he watches from that height "the inevitable mass-disasters" that will affect the rest of us.

Sometimes my friend reminds me of Jeffers—he has had such faith in his body: its strength and flexibility, resilience. Autonomy has come first for him, although, like the rest of us, he both longs for

76

and fears intimacy. After some treatment, he found reasons to free himself from the invasive mechanical intimacy of medicine, drugs and machines. He'll go it alone, a body integrated and intact.

My grandfather, a physician, died from the same illness my friend has now. But my grandfather was in his seventies when the disease showed itself. My friend was in his forties.

My son was one when his disease manifested; now he's eighteen. My intimacy with his body lasted longer than any typical relationship between mother and child. I touched and wiped his face and body as he has had no capacity for self-care. I fed him through a tube, releasing liquid in slow bursts into a port in his abdomen. Now a machine feeds him and his father does the personal care when a nurse does not. I still touch his face and kiss his forehead. I still worry he will die. And this first separation from his body feels like the beginning of grief, a waking recognition of intimate loss.

When my grandfather died, it was my turn in the small room downstairs. He'd been still for hours, snoring almost as he had when vibrantly alive. Then consciousness surfaced and he called hoarsely for my grandmother by her nickname. My grandmother dropped a dishcloth, my mother and her sisters hurried. As I left, I looked back at them circled around his bed, singing. That call to my grandmother was his last breath—I've been certain I was the witness.

After he died, my grandmother sold the camp. She said she could never return. I'd trusted it would always be there. While it was under contract, my cousin and I descended the long stairs to the beach to chip away bits of a large sparkling rock that had been at the center of every game we'd played, its flat surface a bench, a table, a drying rack for bowls and figurines we'd form from the clay a foot beneath the sand. Cutting the rock was a violation, but we felt justified in holding on to what we'd lost. And that may be the nature of grievance: a determination to declaim in perpetuity a relationship irrevocably broken.

I can't find my pieces of Diamond Rock. I'd look for them, but the spot from which we chiseled them has already changed, worn soft by wind, water and sand, while the pieces I would like to grip once more retain their edges. How beautiful and a little terrible.

"These things," Jeffers says, meaning government and interdependence, "are Progress." His poem descends from the sublimity of the mountaintop—because that's what the sublime entails, beauty mixed with terror—to the valley of political grievance. The images give way to cynical rhetoric about civilization: "surely one always knew that cultures decay, and life's end is death." In Jeffers' poetry, human relationships are not connection, they're a reflection of helplessness. Our "vast populations," he writes, are "incapable of free survival." My grandfather trusted ecosystems far more than Jeffers. Only weeds are capable of free survival, and yet weeds may take over the world.

The doctors now call my son "medically fragile," but I think he's no more fragile than all of humankind, at risk of fire, drowning, disease, accidents, sudden death heretofore unknown. Jeffers' "inevitable mass disasters" are nothing more than the fate of any individual body as cells decay, age gathers and disintegration perches on the horizon. Each day "the circle is closed, and the net / Is being hauled in." Some days the seine-net rises to the surface more clearly than others, with fewer or more fish. Myself, I will still trust the great cities, luminous with dependency and information, because doctors in them, for the time being, have saved my son from death. My grandfather never met my son.

My father has said the last of the generation before him has passed. Someday I will say that, as though each tier of my family entwines its own rough netting that sinks out of sight, empty, after hauling the little fish in.

Objects my grandfather gave me came to fill the space left by his death: books inscribed with his spidery handwriting, a pocket knife, a magnifying glass, a necklace. Many people have written many things about grief, enough books to fill a small town's library. I don't want to read any of them. If the dead can't live with me anymore, I want to live with their things.

I worry that if my friend dies, I'll have no object of his to keep, save a few letters. The bulk of our correspondence has been digital, virtual, the way our emotional closeness approximates physical intimacy but has not embodied it.

I wrote a prose poem some years ago from which I've excised these words: "Dawn lifts white-bright film from a lake surface faceted geometric, shimmering mathematic. How the world trickles with uncanny precision through our fingers and how of all things love is most terrible." These should fit into another work, but so far, they don't. Maybe I'll have them chiseled on my gravestone.

My son doesn't speak, read or write. I have no words of his to hold, nothing from the deep water of his consciousness. While I know which of his things he likes, there's no patina of touch on anything he owns. He has no calluses on his hands or feet, even his shoes show no signs of wear. He's the purest being I know; however, I'll let no one make a martyr of his disease or disability, the way Jeffers makes an example of all humankind, *each person in himself helpless, on all dependent*. We've made an effort to steer him from suffering and toward joy. If anything, he's *martyr to a motion not his own*. Roethke.

Sometimes I dream of becoming rich and buying back the camp at any price, but it would never be mine again. Others have inhabited it, made it their own. My grandmother chose to sell it to grieve her own loss. Of my own grievance, I think of Theodore Roethke's love poem to his deceased student, "I, with no rights in this matter, / Neither father nor lover."

There's no grief without grievance, no beauty without terror. No intimacy without longing for autonomy—which is where my friend and I find each other these days: guilty, I yearn for some freedom from my son, he for companionship and love. *I knew a woman,* Roethke wrote, *lovely in her bones:*

What's freedom for? To know eternity.
I swear she cast a shadow white as stone.
But who would count eternity in days?

Life's end is death—we can say it mechanically or lyrically.

Grief, grievance, beauty, terror—these intersect where absolute separation entangles love and hope. The seine-net makes a diamond grid of these knots, the slipping and simultaneous tightening of one line against another.

Trace "martyr" to its source and you find Greek, "witness," a chronicler of existence. *I measure time by how a body sways.* Or waves rolling to the shore. Objects on a shelf for your review. *I still see you as though you were 21,* I tell my friend. I knew my son lovely in his bones.

One more knot on a string of days. *Shanti, shanti, shanti.*

Altimeter

White and blue corrugated tubes joined at a clear, narrow pipe that disappeared into the corner of his mouth and descended invisibly to his lungs. One tube delivered oxygen, the other pumped CO_2 out. Beside the bed, an LED display used black peaks to show where the machine breathed for him, and gray peaks (hardly any) where he drew his own. A suite of machines against the wall administered, variously, medications, IV fluids, or formula, while others monitored vital signs. Tubes and leads were everywhere, and a big strip of white tape ran under his nose to secure the breathing tube, a strange elongated mustache. His eyes were closed.

All winter Robert, my son, had been sick—coughing, a wet cough. Though illness and complications were nothing new with him, somewhere in the back of my mind, a little bell rang. I took him to his gastroenterologist, who ordered an x-ray, which revealed his Nissen fundoplication, a stomach surgery to control acid reflux, had slipped, loosened, herniated.

Exploratory probes were the next step: endoscopy (esophagus and stomach) and bronchoscopy (lungs). Robert was placed under general anesthesia and intubated. After Dr. R found a rapidly worsening pneumonia, Robert failed extubation, a plain way of saying that when the ventilator used during anesthesia was removed, he couldn't breathe on his own. He was literally drowning in his secretions.

When I saw Robert next, he was intubated under paralytic sedation, the ventilator gently inflating and deflating his lungs: a machine keeping my child alive.

That was the first failed extubation.

It's tempting to analogize body and machine: the heart a pump, the lungs a bellows, the stomach a churn, the brain a computer, as if we could forever make these organs function. Bodies are never machines—they lack the precision, hard edges, durability. We are a collection of specialized cells, each with its job to do, each cell fallible, each with a number of others at the ready until too many fail. Cells like lemmings into the breach, biochemical processes firing away

81

both under control and independent of the brain in patterns barely understood. The skin holds together a teeming congress working under threat of dissolution.

—

I saw the Blackbird the day after Phoebe Snow, the singer, died. I never knew devotion to her disabled daughter had caused her disappearance in the 1970s from the music scene. Snow's husband left and she spent the years marshaling resources to care for Valerie. Child, then mother died, four years apart.

The Udvar-Hazy Center is glass, metal pipe and sharp angles clutching the outline of an aircraft hangar. My daughter and I were late for a special science night, so we seemed harried as the guard performed a requisite check of my purse. *Walk down that hall to a set of stairs,* he said, *And you'll find your group near the Blackbird.* I expressed some uncertainty about this Blackbird, and he smiled, *You can't miss it—it doesn't look like any plane you've ever seen.*

The steps served as a look-out over the expanse of planes and space craft scattered over the vast floor or hanging by steel threads from the ceiling. Children reached the height of these aviation wheels, atop which perched planes like birds of prey.

The Blackbird was, in fact, black, and of an unusual shape. At its front wheel, two docents gave a presentation about pitch, roll, and yaw. My daughter asked questions. I stood in awe of this giant black plane, which, up close, seemed to be composed of multiple plates with a grayish cast, from afar an illusion *creation ex nihilo.*

Its nose cone drew to a point and the point extended into space like a probe or needle. The cockpit was a glass triangle tucked into the upward curve from the nose cone, and the plane's undulating outline resembled a cat I could stroke with two hands from the sides of the face and back along the body. Alongside the aircraft, an edge drawn out like a pucker passed for wings as though someone had gently flattened pursed lips. I stood in front and the plane nearly disappeared, save for two huge engines like testicles at the rear.

This spy plane flew at three times the speed of sound and could travel from DC to LA in 64 minutes. A pilot needing to turn would begin preparation 200 to 300 miles in advance.

My trepidation about war and violence aside, I found this awesome, in every permutation of that word from contemporary to Biblical. What did it take to climb into that cockpit and turn this plane's nose down the runway? Would the plane fly me, or I the plane, my hands gripping its controls, fusion of woman and metal—no, a complex glass and metal object formed by other human hands—while the forces of gravity, torsion and acceleration threatened to reduce us to scrap. How exhilarating, this breaking free, while some equal and opposite force pinned me to my seat.

During the first year of Robert's disabilities, I'd watched a bio pic about Oscar Wilde. Consigned to forced labor for his "perversion," Wilde's only joy is writing. He learns, docile, to set his pen down when time is called and his materials whisked away. The film terrified me because I understood my future. For years I would live watching the clock as time drew near, or abandon what I was doing for days due to circumstances—all with an understanding that this would not be temporary.

I once told my daughter that part of running is learning to manage your breath. Part of caregiving is learning to manage constraint, how to pace yourself within its boundaries.

—

We sat in the family lounge, TV chattering softly in the background as Dr. R and Dr. C (the surgeon) explained the erroneous simplicity of our belief that a repair to Robert's Nissen fundoplication would restore him to us. Nissen "revisions," he said, had only a 40 percent success rate. Because Robert had, perhaps, a 50 percent chance (or less) of surviving such a complex surgery due to his pneumonia, the mathematics of the situation were clear. And the gastrointestinal tract—this wrapping of the stomach around the esophagus and stitching it in place—would never tolerate the stress and scar tissue of a third Nissen. If we attempted, if he survived that operation, that extra chance at life would never be available again.

Dr. C was French and his slight accent had initially given my husband and myself the impression of a diplomatic summit—as though we could negotiate the terms of Robert's return to the land of the living. Dr R took my arm and said, carefully, that Robert might not survive this hospitalization at all.

Throughout our discussion, my mind had blacked out intermittently, then blinked on again. Any further thinking seemed out of the question. Before nothingness took me, I sobbed openly in front of doctors, which I'd never done before.

Our conversation took place while the intensive care team tried to extubate Robert. We had had to leave the room. That Robert might not be extubated successfully hadn't occurred to me—at first, the attending physician stepped in to express cautious optimism that Robert was breathing on his own, next to apologize for speaking too soon. He was drowning once again, then back to paralytic sedation and the ventilator. Our meeting broke up.

That was the second failed extubation.

Pretend you're a dragon, I'd said before the endoscopy and bronchoscopy. The best kind to be is the benevolence-breathing dragon, whose smoky light-blue exhalation makes right again whatever it touches. So Robert had gone into his procedure thinking about flying over the world, fixing car accidents and blown-down houses and how everyone would cheer when they saw him coming.

When the second extubation failed, I resorted to pleading with doctors that I'd promised him he would wake up.

—

Once, my daughter asked me where the phrase, "Houston, we have a problem," had come from. She thought Houston was a person.

I told her about the Apollo 13 mission: malfunction in the space ship, repairs solved by mission control with the materials on board the craft, computations done by slide rule, the looming concern the ship and its crew might be irretrievable.

The astronauts were, of course, focused on survival, yet the geometrical curvature of their rescue, a slingshot maneuver around the moon itself, brought them close enough to the object of their desire (a walk on its surface) that its necessary sacrifice burrowed into their hearts.

Neil Armstrong had walked on the moon. Our kindergarten teacher gave us each a commemorative Apollo 11 stamp. It was summer and we watched the moon landing from the television in my parents' bedroom. *One small step for man.* Black and white TV images and the world in bloom outside our windows. "Here" evaporated into a screen, cathode tube and wires. *One giant leap for mankind.*

When the space capsules from various missions approached earth, Walter Cronkite broadcast conversation from the cockpit: military jokes, calm and cool voices of astronauts giving the impression that all this was routine. Just the way military men on bases where my dad did summer duty—Fort Belvoir, Fort Lee—had been solemn and funny at the same time.

Then Cronkite's voice and those of reporters got tense as the capsule hit outer layers of the stratosphere and entered radio blackout as the last piece of the big rocket, what was left after its long voyage and the intermittent jettison of its parts, hit the friction of what we called air. Would the heat shields hold? Atmosphere slowed the capsule's speed, flames dragging at its convex base, as friction threatened to break those panels apart.

Silence. Silence. Waiting and cameras were trained at the sky, at the place the capsule should emerge into blue of air just before hitting blue of ocean. And cameras panned the sky again. Then a black dot and bigger and it was the capsule and a big parachute deployed. And then voices.

Robert had had anesthesia often—going under, either through a mask or, sometimes, the agent delivered through his g-tube. The white sheet under him, bright lights, anesthesiologist explaining what would happen, that the anesthesia smelled like bubble gum. And his startled face each and every time as the mask covered his mouth and nose. Breathing, then his breath held, startled, and breathing again. Eyes wide in alarm and then drooping closed.

How quickly they made me leave each time when I'd wanted to linger one second longer.

Then, his return. Limbs and eyes stirring, he'd wake to remember, then again not know where he was or had been.

One afternoon, I was pulled through a CT scan repeatedly, the room quiet, white and cold. And big. Because the equipment was big. And lonely because the technician left the room to monitor computers behind a glass wall.

Just me entering the machine's white ring, wondering if my elbows resting by my ears would hit. The recorded voice told me to breathe in, hold my breath. Cooperate. Long pause. The whirring whine of whatever made the images and my trying not to look below the little sign because it said, do not look into the red square. But the sign didn't explain why.

Then the recorded voice said again, with odd urgency for a machine, *breathe!*

———

Over the next few days, the room remained peaceful, Robert in a light coma, the machine and its dark and light peaks. I had my feet up on the bed, reading a book. The ventilator was adjusted periodically to see how much Robert could breathe on his own and for how long. Then the doctors eased his sedation.

Time came to remove the tube again—the third, last time they would try. The doctors let us stay and we were pressed to the edge of the room as the team circled his bed—two intensive care nurses, the attending, a resident, a respiratory therapist.

Tunnel vision—the choreographed pull of the vent tube, longer than I would have suspected, Robert coughing gasping choking, his eyes wide. The nurses talking reassuringly while suctioning fluids from his mouth and trachea. The attending issuing instructions, the respiratory therapist manipulating machines. Gasp and choke, the sedation lifted so he would be conscious while body and machine separated. I bit my lower lip, but never closed my eyes, calling encouragement to him.

Robert at the center, others on the periphery working fast and competently. All of it the way the delivery room becomes active, suddenly, after hours of solitude, when it's time to push. Outside myself watching this birth—that struggle to breathe what it means to be alive, from the physiological to the metaphysical.

The third extubation was successful.

—

The next day, I felt like Sam Shepard playing Chuck Yeager in *The Right Stuff* with the plane wreck of my life burning in the background as I walked toward whatever constituted civilization, my face singed and carrying what was left of my parachute.

Yeager, unauthorized, takes the jet down the runway for one reason: to see how high it can be flown, the jet's nose rising in silence, up and up, so high the altimeter cracks and g-forces push Yeager back against the seat while he struggles to stay conscious.

An obvious analogy: Icarus. What was his cause of death? The burning of the borrowed wings? His head-long plunge into the sea? Or did he fly so high the air thinned, compressing his body and his lungs so that he could not breathe?

Pushing the jet as far as its mechanics will allow: the altimeter will break and the sleek beauty of the aircraft will stall at first just so quietly and then pitch into a flat spin—the horizon here and then gone again—all I will hear will be the sound of my own breath in my ears.

In the film the plane spins in silence, Yeager's body ejects, the seat bottom rising away from the camera, and for long minutes, the plane dives toward the pale brown and green surface of the planet, and we think Yeager will survive but we don't know.

The gastroenterologist made a special visit to Robert's hospital room at the end of a long day during which, I am sure, she saw dozens of patients, performed various surgical procedures, and was probably ready to go home. Instead, she sat wearily down opposite where I sat with my feet propped on Robert's bed. My son ignored his doctor the way 16-year-olds resist authority, staring at the television.

Dr R asked how I was doing, and I remember the faint gray

light in the room. We were still in the intensive care unit, but most of the machines had been removed so it was quieter than it had been. I'd moved from numb shock to my usual sense that we'd made it through another crisis and the world would return to its usual routines.

I liked Dr R very much, but I had never seen her, a person quite frank and to the point in all her dealings—diminutive in stature, but not in presence—never seen her quite so frank and to the point. "Mrs. Stone," she said, "this is not going back to normal. You are used to the idea that it can," she explained, "because you've taken such scrupulously good care of Robert all this time, all these years. Most children with his level of disability and medical fragility are in and out of the hospital like this all the time."

In other words, she grabbed me by my psychic shoulders and she shook some sense into me. Or thought she had.

By then, engines had already pushed me off the tarmac, firing asphalt to tar, metal wings bearing the negative and positive pressures that keep a jet aloft—and shock waves were behind me, even if turbulence roiled ahead.

The Chaos
for Mary Shelley

1997 :
I bid my hideous progeny go forth
and prosper. I have an affection for it,
for it was the offspring of happy days
when death and grief were but words
which found no true echo in my heart : M.S., 1831

Anxiety cupboard of suburbia : houses gestational pods
        daddies scatter for work in suits and ties

mommies push strollers to the park : daddies return
        sometimes it is dark : sometimes light

it depends on the season : close the door on your unnecessary fears

      Natura nihil agit frustra, is the onely indisputable axiome in Philosophy

The heart comes first always : beats within the lump projected
        on the screen : later the face before bones thicken

so a face recognizable (this is the one for whom I would lie down
        and die) : strobes with a wide-eyed skull

        There are no Grotesques in nature nor anything framed
          to fill up empty cantons, and unnecessary spaces

The delivery room is like this : light & dark : dark & shadows
        tightening & relaxing pain crenellating then : easing

the room white brilliants shatter peripheral: forced through barriers
        love comes : eerily like God's breath

his beauty a barricade : behind it crouches something aware

1998 :
Dream that my little baby came
to life again—that it had only been cold & that
we rubbed it before the fire & it lived : M.S., 1815

June the Pacific his feet balance on

packed sand the tide undermines

thrill of fear as water surges

last snapshot framed icon

August a hospital puppet body

punctured digitized monitored

(ask the wisp inside to stay)

his cry measured, repetitive

Resignation defeat an end

to invention : reality nimbler past this

not what we made but what

love in its making requires

whom we truley love like our owne selves, wee forget their lookes,
nor can our memory retaine the Idea of their faces; and it is
no wonder, for they are our selves, and affection
makes their lookes our owne

1999 :
*Invention does not consist in creating out of
a void, but out of chaos—it can give form to dark,
shapeless substances, but cannot bring into being
the substance itself* : M.S., 1816

Summer on Lake Geneva Percy

    Byron's laughter off waves in bursts

        sail inflated deflated inflated

            (a human heart tacking)

          Rain dragged evening sheeting

       toward the manse at its hearth

    flames groped hands clasped mind

dilating upon an idea so hideous

Winter forced lungs full of fluid

     constellated stars held back

        the void yet in chaos cellular

          a spark tindered necessity vanity

In briefe, we are all monsters, that is, a composition of man and beast

2000:
There is no deformity but in monstrosity,
wherein notwithstanding there is a kind of beauty,
Nature so ingeniously contriving those irregular parts,
* as they become sometimes more remarkable*
* than the principal Fabrick :* Browne, *Religio Medici,* 1643

My heart is a cupboard filled with love and fear : doors snap
        open and birds flock out : black pressure rising throngs

a thousand childish vees : half-hearts bursting
        as around us small perfect bodies skip a beat while

Victor has pushed and pushed his dogs : sled's runners slicing
        rust slough behind them gasping : cold

air burning down : acid air wrenching up blood
        exertion : brains flame against the polar ice while

Clara : William : Percy—dead—1818 : 1819 : 1822
        blue tongues : fevered pores : the brain shuts down

on the sight of blinking lights on shore : or
        a face framed with damp black hair while

                    to speake yet more narrowly, there was never anything
                                ugly, or mis-shapen, but the Chaos

ahead of all, the monster leaps nimbly
from floe to floe shrieking
a falsetto promise
to burn himself
alive

Notes

"Winter Kept Us Warm"

Title comes from a passage in T.S. Eliot's *The Waste Land*: "Winter kept us warm, covering / Earth in forgetful snow, feeding / A little life with dried tubers."

"The Brain as Variation"

David Antin quotations from his mixed genre piece "talking at blérancourt," which appears in his collection *i never knew what time it was*.

"And So Love Any Thing"

Samplings from Theodore Roethke's poem, "I Knew a Woman," and John Peele's poem, "What Thing is Love?" Not all quotations or adapted quotations are italicized.

"Death Valley, California"

Samplings from John Donne's poem, "A Nocturnall upon St. Lucies Day, being the shortest day"; reference to Oppenheimer's response to first atomic bomb test (he quoted the Bhagavad Gita: "Now I am become Death, the destroyer of worlds").

"Notes on Creativity & Originality"

David Foster Wallace quotation from his essay, "The Nature of the Fun"; Crick & Watson anecdote from James D. Watson's memoir, *The Double Helix*; "art is life distilled" a reference to Gwendolyn Brooks' remark that "poetry is life distilled."

For more information on the relationship of Renaissance faculty psychology to "invention" and the five parts of rhetoric, see Frances Yates' *The Art of Memory*. For more on the semantic evolution of "genius" and "originality," see the preface to Edward Tayler's anthology, *Literary Criticism of 17th Century England*. For background on Renaissance ideas about sex and sexuality, see Thomas Laqueur's *Making Sex: Body and Gender from the Greeks to Freud*.

"Disability & Space-Time Considerations"

The 14-story building and baseball analogies are from Gary Zukav's *The Dancing Wu-Li Masters: An Overview of the New Physics*. Physicist quotations from the film documentary *Particle Fever:* physicist one, Nima Arkani-Hamed (Princeton University); physicist two, Savas Dimopoulos (Stanford University). For more on the behavior of light and particles, as well as the Higgs bosun/celebrity analogy, watch physicist Brian Greene's PBS series, *NOVA: The Fabric of the Cosmos*.

This essay responds to the question posed to scientists in *Particle Fever:* "Why study physics, rather than ...?" Finally, on the grounds of CERN (The European Organization for Nuclear Research) at which the LHC is located, there's a metal sculpture of Lord Shiva.

"Life As We Know It"

Samplings adapted from Alfred, Lord Tennyson's poem, "Ulysses," not all of which are italicized.

"Meiosis"

Samplings adapted from William Wordsworth's poem, "Ode: Intimations of Immortality," not all of which are italicized.

"Tomb of the Unknown"

Arlington Cemetery statistics from the National Park Service's official website (http://www.arlingtoncemetery.mil/#/); a common citation: 3 billion nucleotides of human DNA would fill one million pages (250 pp. = average book), for examples, see the educational resources of the Human Genome Project at https://www.genome.gov/10001772/all-about-the—human-genome-project-hgp/.

"Grief"

Lake Champlain data from Lake Champlain Land Trust: http://www.lclt.org/about-lake-champlain/lake-champlain-facts/; various word definitions from Merriam-Webster online; "I with no rights in this matter …" is from Theodore Roethke's poem "Elegy for Jane (My student thrown by a horse)"; the remaining Roethke quotations are from his poem "I Knew a Woman."

"Altimeter"

Films referenced: *Wilde* (1997); *The Right Stuff* (1983).

"The Chaos"

Mary Shelley quotations from the 1831 preface to *Frankenstein* and her diary; Thomas Browne quotations from *Religio Medici* (The Religion of a Doctor). *Natura nihil agit frustra* translates as "Nature does nothing in vain."

Jeneva Burroughs Stone has published poetry and essays in many literary journals, including *The Colorado Review, Poetry International, Los Angeles Review of Books,* and *Pleiades.* Her work in nonfiction has been honored with fellowships from the MacDowell and Millay Colonies. She holds an MFA from the Warren Wilson Program for Writers, a PhD from Columbia University, and a BA from Middlebury College.

Jeneva does volunteer work for Rare Genomics Institute and CareGifted, the first dedicated to helping families of undiagnosed children find answers, the second to long-term caregiver respite. She is also a contributing editor to *Pentimento: Journal of All Things Disability*, which is dedicated to promoting the voices of caregivers and writers with disabilities. She lives in Bethesda, Maryland.

A Note on the Type

The interior typeface is Adobe Garamond Pro, designed by Robert Slimbach in 1989 as an interpretation of original roman and italic faces by the French type designers Claude Garamond (1505-1561) and Robert Granjon (1530-1590).

About Phoenicia Publishing

Phoenicia Publishing is an independent press based in Montreal but involved, through a network of online connections, with writers and artists all over the world. We are interested in words and images that illuminate culture, spirit, and the human experience. A particular focus is on writing and art about travel between cultures— whether literally, through lives of refugees, immigrants, and travelers, or more metaphorically and philosophically—with the goal of enlarging our understanding of one another through universal and particular experiences of change, displacement, disconnection, assimilation, sorrow, gratitude, longing and hope.

We are committed to the innovative use of the web and digital technology in all aspects of publishing and distribution, and to making high-quality works available that might not be viable for larger publishers. We work closely with our authors, and are pleased to be able to offer them a greater share of royalties than is normally possible.

Your support of this endeavor is greatly appreciated.

Our complete catalogue is online at www.phoeniciapublishing.com

Made in the USA
Middletown, DE
07 December 2016